THE 25 DAY | AYURVEDA CLEANSE

A Holistic Wellness Plan Using Ayurvedic Practices to Reset Your Health Naturally

KERRY HARLING

Certified Ayurvedic Practitioner & Founder of The Holistic Highway

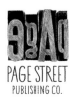

PAGE STREET
PUBLISHING CO.

PAGE STREET
PUBLISHING CO.

First published in 2019 by
Page Street Publishing Co.
27 Congress Street, Suite 105
Salem, MA 01970
www.pagestreetpublishing.com

Distributed by Macmillan, sales in Canada by The Canadian Manda Group.

22   21   20   19   1   2   3   4

ISBN-13: 978-1-62414-835-4

ISBN-10: 1-62414-835-2

Library of Congress Control Number: 2019931253

Cover and book design by Sara Pollard and Meg Baskis for Page Street Publishing Co.

Food photography by Toni Zernik

Pages 2 & 3: © Shutterstock/Mooshny, page 5: © Shutterstock/Zdenka Darula, pages 5 & 17: © Shutterstock/Maridav, cover and page 10: © Shutterstock/Evgeny Atamanenko, page 18: © Shutterstock/Soloviova Liudmyla, page 21: © Shutterstock/everst, page 31: © Shutterstock/etorres, page 32: © Shutterstock/Fortyforks, page 33: © Shutterstock/paulynn, page 108: © Shutterstock/George Rudy, page 113: © Shutterstock/ZephyrMedia, page 114: © Shutterstock/Julia Sudnitskaya, page 120: © Shutterstock/Alliance, page 121: © Shutterstock/JPC-PROD, page 136: © Shutterstock/imtmphoto, page 144: © Shutterstock/Pressmaster, cover and page 170: © Shutterstock/jesadaphorn, page 175: © Shutterstock/billnoll, page 212: © Shutterstock/Kite_rin

Yoga Illustrations by Bitsy McCann

Printed and bound in the United States

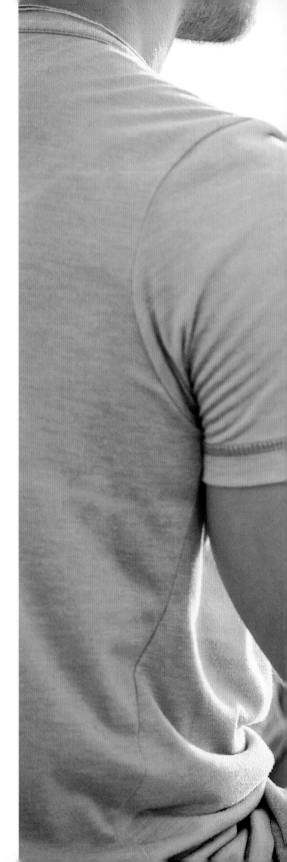

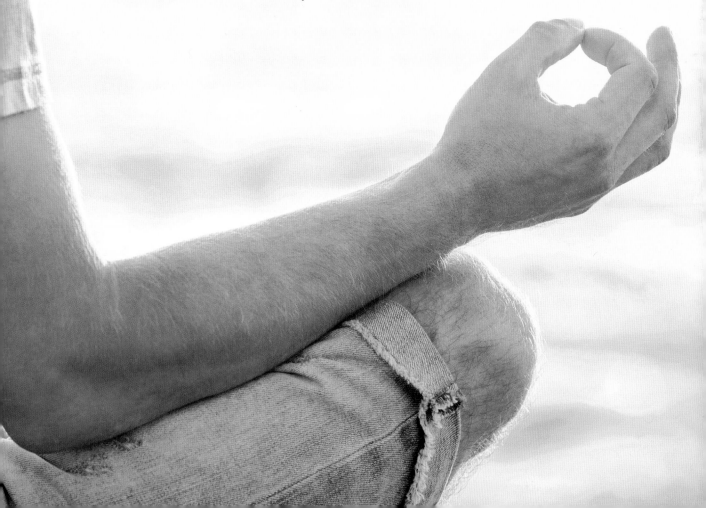

DEDICATION

To my mother, who was my first inspiration and whose unconditional love I carry in this life.

To my sister, who always inspires me, shares that love and is my best friend.

To my son, who will pass on that inspiration and unconditional love to generations I may not see.

To you, who inspire me every day with your willingness to try a new way, a new path and a new direction.

And finally, to the great scholars of Ayurveda, Charaka and Sushruta, who allow us to embrace Ayurveda in this modern world.

CONTENTS

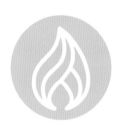
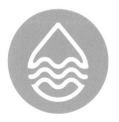

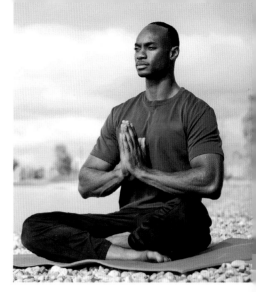

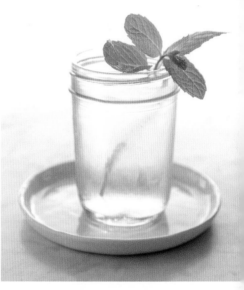

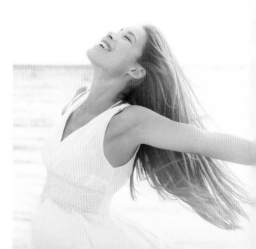

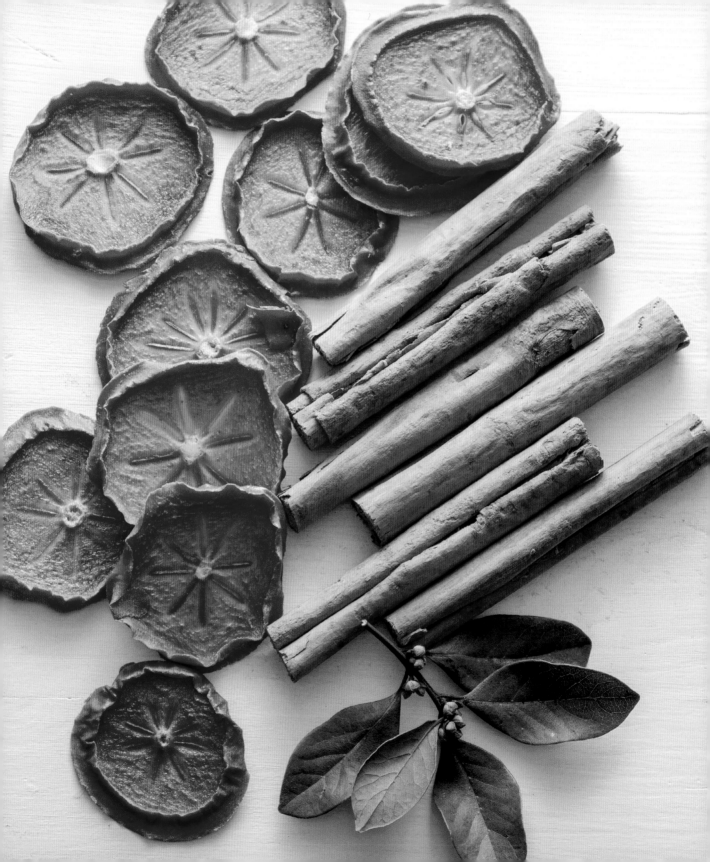

FOREWORD

From a Skeptic's Point of View

My name is Justin Timlin, and I am the author's son and co-owner of the Holistic Highway. I am also a natural Ayurveda skeptic. In fact, I'd never even heard of it until five years ago. Shocked?

I'm here to give you a perspective on Ayurveda that most people can't give. It's the view from someone who owns an Ayurveda business, yet is not a practitioner or a converted follower.

This business started with my mother, Kerry Harling, sharing her Ayurveda training and skills with family and friends and trying to help them in any way she could. At the time, I didn't really understand what my mom was doing. However, she was incredibly passionate about this thing called "Ayurveda," and when she asked me to help out, I dutifully obliged. As a brand and marketing strategist, I simply did some of the things I usually do for my clients, and I was just helping out my mom. Out of this limited partnership, the Holistic Highway was born.

My background is in hard science and business. I have a neuroscience degree from the University of Massachusetts and an MBA from Georgetown University. I am a man grounded by logic, reason, science and empirical evidence. I raised an eyebrow at things like cleanses and doshas and thought they weren't real science. That is, until I saw firsthand the results the Ayurveda cleanse and system of medicine had on people.

After five years behind the scenes, I can tell you without a doubt that Ayurveda works. And the reason it works is so shockingly simple! Ayurveda recognizes that we are all unique and that there is no one size fits all. There is no one diet that suits all people, no one type of exercise, one supplement or lifestyle change. What is right for me might not be right for you. After all, we live different lives, have different careers, live in different environments and have different genetics.

Modern health care, with its amazing technological advances, skilled surgeons and life-saving pharmaceuticals, has failed in its core promise: to keep us well! Our system of medicine has siloed and has had to specialize and subspecialize to such an extent that we no longer see the whole person.

That's where the Holistic Highway is different. As part of the University of Pittsburgh's Center for Integrative Medicine, we often work with Western doctors to develop health and wellness plans that integrate Ayurvedic principles of personalization, partnership and prevention with modern technology. The Ayurveda cleanse in this book is one of the powerful tools we use to get people back on the right track to great health.

I've seen firsthand the incredible transformation our clients have had by making simple, sustainable changes to their diet and lifestyle. Combine this with ongoing support and accountability and you, too, can experience this recipe for success. And that's where this book shines.

For those of you on the fence about the effectiveness of an Ayurveda cleanse . . . take it from a skeptic. It works. If you want to know the things you can do right away to start living a healthier, happier lifestyle, this book is the perfect place to start.

In good health,

—Justin Timlin

INTRODUCTION
Not Your Everyday Cleanse

We have reached a tipping point moment in our health. I see it on the streets, in our playgrounds, reflected in our statistics and in my practice. We are a world of sick people. Obesity is a problem in all developed nations, as is diabetes, hypertension, metabolic syndrome and cancer. I see younger and younger children being medicated for anxiety, depression and an inability to focus. I hear the despair in my clients' voices as they complain of a losing battle with weight gain, insomnia, low sex drive and fatigue. More and more people in my practice have spent years on medications for a countless number of these and other issues. And lastly, the incidence and prevalence of autoimmune diseases such as Hashimoto's thyroiditis, celiac disease, rheumatoid arthritis and ulcerative colitis have increased significantly over the last thirty years.

What are we doing wrong? We have forgotten to live right . . . to be part of nature. To eat seasonally and engage in a lifestyle that is individually right for us. We have forgotten to slow down and marvel at the world around us, and we have forgotten how to exercise the right way. We are out of balance!

The daily rigors of life today create tremendous stress on our bodies and take a serious toll on our health. This problem is compounded with unhealthy foods, sedentary careers and a culture of medicine that treats the symptoms and not the underlying causes. And sometimes it takes a wake-up call—and sadly, for many of us, that wake-up call is an illness. You know, like when the body says, "I can't do this anymore" and just throws in the towel.

My body threw in the towel.

I spent most of my life unhealthy and chronically fatigued. This always surprises people when I tell them, considering my profession, but I spent years being diagnosed with a myriad of diseases, including fibromyalgia, depression, Lyme disease, anxiety and chronic fatigue. I was taking medication for all of them.

I would go to the doctor and be prescribed the latest drug for my latest symptoms. No one tried to understand the underlying cause of my health problems. As a single mother, working full-time and with a rambunctious young son, I couldn't afford to be sick. Life was stressful enough without constantly being ill and exhausted. I was sick and tired of being sick and tired, and I was desperate. It was at this point in my life that I turned to an alternative health practitioner. I was diagnosed with mercury toxicity. Finally, I knew the cause of all my problems! I could at last be healthy once and for all!

Not so fast.

Five years of treatment left me mercury free, but I was still lacking the energy and vitality of a younger, healthier me. The reason for this is because I had only solved half the equation. I fixed the underlying cause of my problems, but I hadn't changed my lifestyle to maintain my health. I was still living the same way I had been my entire life—the same way that helped make me sick in the first place. I was still out of balance.

It was at this time that I was introduced to Ayurveda, a 5,000-year-old system of medicine with its roots in India that treats each person as unique and balances the body, mind and soul. I learned I was fatigued because my *agni* (digestive fire) was too low and I had built up *ama* (toxins). So, I underwent an Ayurveda cleansing process. Just one month later, I found my vitality and energy improving. It was amazing!

I was so absolutely astounded by the power of this simple yet effective method of health that I made a major life change. I decided to study Ayurveda so I could help others discover the incredible way this avenue of health could improve their lives, like it did mine.

As an educator, I decided to give back in the best way I knew how: by teaching others. It is not enough to give you a solution for a day; I give you the knowledge to achieve great health for your entire life. And in this book, I will give you the tools needed in order to feel full of vitality, energy and happiness every day for the rest of your life.

The Ayurveda cleanse is the perfect way to start looking at your life and your health differently.

WHAT THIS BOOK CAN DO FOR YOU

By following this cleanse, you will start a new way of living and eating that will benefit you. Your goal may be weight loss, or you may wish to understand how food can heal or maybe you're done with waking up sick and tired. Whatever your personal goal, I will be right by your side, as this cleanse was written for *you*. It will ignite your digestive fire so you can reduce the accumulation of toxins, which are causing your symptoms.

The cleanse is broken down into three phases:

- Phase 1 is the prep and pre-cleanse.
- Phase 2 is the heart of the cleanse.
- Phase 3 is the post-cleanse.

Each phase has a day-by-day schedule, a section on yoga poses, pranayama (breathwork), journal prompts to help you detox emotionally and lots of delicious recipes to try.

So, curl up on the couch, make yourself some detox tea and let's dive right into the cleanse so you can start on your path to health and vitality.

TESTIMONIALS

"This program was so much easier to follow than I thought it would be. I was expecting it to be a struggle like every diet I tried in the past, but I loved it and have completely changed my lifestyle for the better. It has opened up a whole new phase of my life!"

—Roberta Kashalk, California

"I'm making my health a priority and people are noticing a difference in me already. The small, daily Ayurvedic practices are leading to significant shifts!"

—Shawn Marie Rehold, Washington

"I don't really know what you did to me, but I can honestly say that it is the first time in a long trail of dieting where my mind is set more on the process than on the end result and where I am really looking for a permanent change in lifestyle rather than on just losing some weight quickly and then getting back to the old habits. So, thank you for that. Yes, it is a bit challenging, but it's also fun discovering new tastes and foods as well as a new will I did not know I had."

—Raluca Gabriela, Bucharest, Romania

"After listening to Kerry and doing some research, I decided to give myself a birthday present that would change my life. I became one of Kerry's clients, and I started her cleanse. I lost a total of 11 pounds (4.9 kg)! This was amazing to me because I never felt hungry. I was not dieting; I was eating the right foods to help me restart my digestion and help me burn fat. And the best part, I feel SO good. I am so looking forward to learning this new lifestyle and all it has to offer. This was the best birthday present I ever gave to myself."

—Fran Spine, New Jersey

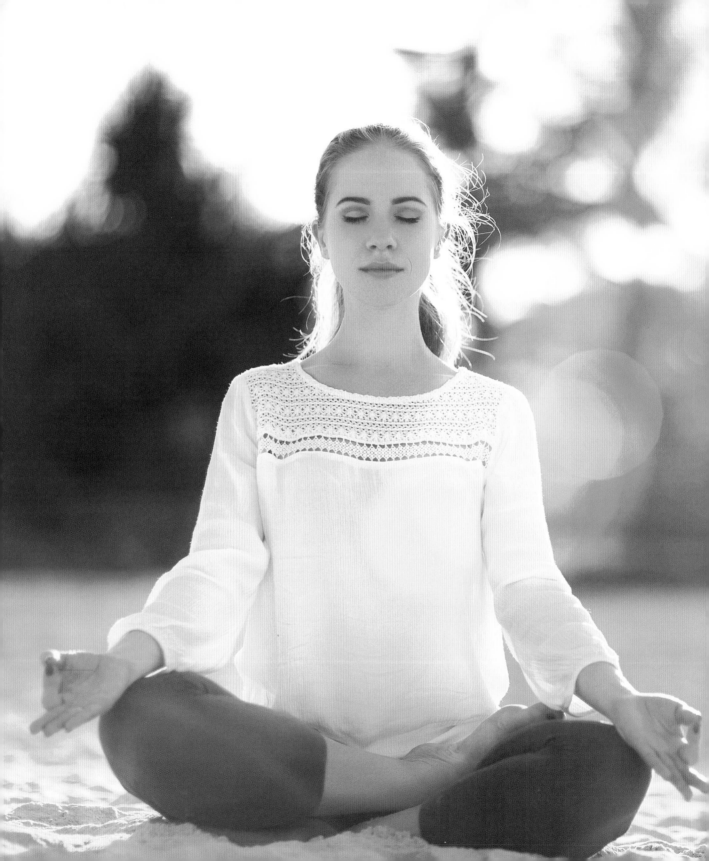

Chapter 1

THE AYURVEDA HEALING SYSTEM

Ayurveda is based on the following principles:

- **There is no "one size fits all."** There is no one drug that suits all people, no one diet, exercise regimen, supplement or lifestyle change.

- **Food is medicine.** We can unlock the power of food to heal disease and achieve optimal health.

- **Foods should change with the seasons.** Each season is associated with different elements and foods that will strengthen your health.

- **Like increases like and opposites balance.** Take in the opposite qualities through the five senses. This brings balance.

- **You are what you digest.** You may know the old saying, "You are what you eat," but I'd like to add to that and say, "You are what you digest and absorb!" In my practice, I frequently see people complaining of fatigue, brain fog, anxiety and depression. Often, they are eating a very clean diet, but they haven't seen improvement because they aren't able to digest and absorb all the great vitamins and minerals they are consuming.

- **Nutrition is anything we take in through the five senses.** By using the input of all our senses, we create pathways whereby we ingest all the qualities of the world and form our perceptions. Our perceptions depend upon nurturing those senses, which in turn nurture our health.

- **Health is holistic.** The definition of health from the World Health Organization (WHO) is: "Health is a well-balanced mind, a well-formed body and good elimination." When the doshas (metabolic types, page 12) are in balance and the mind and body are in harmony, health naturally follows.

WHAT MAKES AN AYURVEDA CLEANSE DIFFERENT?

This 25-day Ayurveda cleanse is designed to "clean out" your current digestion, ridding you of ama (page 22), which are digestive toxins that can lead to gas, bloating, fatigue, diarrhea, heartburn, stiff or achy joints, heaviness, brain fog and lethargy. The cleanse does this by working with your dosha (metabolic type, page 12), and in turn, fires up your digestive fire or agni (page 22) so that the effects of an Ayurveda cleanse are transformative. Typical benefits include improved skin, sleep, digestion, energy and mental clarity along with a reduction in bloating, constipation, headaches and joint pain.

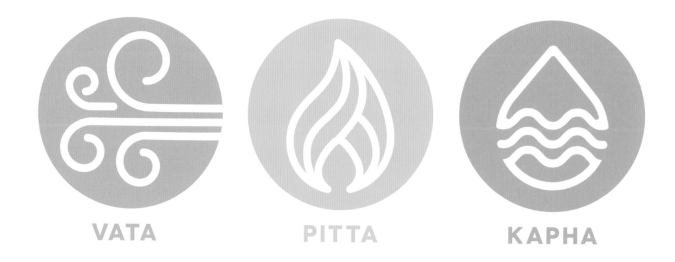

VATA   **PITTA**   **KAPHA**

As you get started on your cleanse to reset your health and life, we begin with an understanding of how you are going to return vitality to your body by using food as medicine. Part of this lesson entails busting myths that circulate around the nutrition world today, and another part involves you figuring out through some fun and simple quizzes which metabolic type (dosha) you are, so you can then maximize the rewards of the Ayurveda cleanse.

This cleanse works because it is customized based on your dosha.

SO, WHAT'S A DOSHA, DARLING?

Ayurveda is a constitutional-based system of medicine that classifies people into three categories. These categories have specific physical, emotional and mental qualities that are determined at conception. These three constitutional types, or doshas, are *Vata*, *Pitta* and *Kapha*. Your body is a combination of all three doshas.

Doshas create balance in our bodies, and when they go out of balance, they create symptoms and ultimately, disease. While all of us have Vata, Pitta and Kapha in us, we have them in unique proportions. That is what makes each of us uniquely different.

Which Dosha Are You?

Have you ever wondered why some people are upbeat and happy while others always see the glass as half empty? How come some people worry incessantly and others take adversity in stride? Why can your friend eat cakes, cookies, breads and snacks in abundance, whereas you only have to look at a pastry to gain five pounds (2.3 kg)?

The key to these answers lies in your dosha. Just as you are born with a unique genetic makeup, you are also born with a unique proportion of doshas. These doshas determine your individual temperament and physical characteristics. They are made up of the five elements: air, space, water, fire and earth. When the doshas are out of balance, they cause physical and mental symptoms. Determining your dominant dosha or doshas and keeping them in balance is the key to maintaining your health and personalizing your cleanse.

Take the dosha quiz starting on the next page to find out what your dominant dosha is. Some of the characteristics will resonate with you; others you will see in your family and friends. Become familiar with your dosha so you can better understand you!

Dosha Questionnaire*

1. For each category, please circle the option that best describes you. (If you feel you can equally relate to more than one of the descriptions, circle all that apply.)

2. When taking the questionnaire, select the description that best fits how you most recently are—within the past few weeks.

3. After finishing a profile: For each column, tally up how many descriptions you circled. This number goes in the Subtotal row at the bottom of each profile.

4. After finishing the profiles, record all your profile totals in the Totals Chart.

5. Note the column you have the most points in, and then find the corresponding dosha type following the questionnaire.

Mental Profile

Category	VATA	PITTA	KAPHA
Mental activity	Quick mind, restless	Sharp intellect, aggressive	Calm, steady, stable
Memory	Short-term best	Good general memory	Long-term best
Thoughts	Constantly changing	Fairly steady	Steady, stable, fixed
Concentration	Short-term focus best	Better than average mental concentration	Good ability for long-term focus
Ability to learn	Quick grasp of learning	Medium to moderate grasp	Slow to learn new things
Dreams	Fearful, flying, running, jumping	Angry, fiery, violent, adventurous	Include water, clouds, relationships, romance
Sleep	Interrupted, light	Sound, medium	Sound, heavy, long
Speech	Fast, sometimes missing words	Fast, sharp, clear-cut	Slow, clear, sweet
Voice	High pitch	Medium pitch	Low pitch
Mental subtotal:	_____	_____	_____

Used with permission from Dr. John Douillard, DC, CAP, of https://lifespa.com.

Behavioral Profile

Category	VATA	PITTA	KAPHA
Eating speed	Quick	Medium	Slow
Hunger level	Irregular	Sharp, need food when hungry	Can easily miss meals
Food and drink	Prefers warm	Prefers cold	Prefers dry and warm
Achieving goals	Easily distracted	Focused and driven	Slow and steady
Giving/donations	Gives small amounts	Gives nothing, or large amounts infrequently	Gives regularly and generously
Relationships	Many casual	Intense	Long and deep
Sex drive	Variable or low	Moderate	Strong
Works best	While supervised	Alone	In groups
Weather preference	Aversion to cold	Aversion to heat	Aversion to damp, cool
Reaction to stress	Excites quickly	Medium	Slow to get excited
Financial	Doesn't save, spends quickly	Saves, but big spender	Saves regularly, accumulates wealth
Friendships	Tends toward short-term friendships, makes friends quickly	Tends to be a loner, friends related to occupation	Tends to form long-lasting friendships
Behavioral subtotal:	_____	_____	_____

Emotional Profile

Category	VATA	PITTA	KAPHA
Moods	Change quickly	Change slowly	Steady, unchanging
Reacts to stress with	Fear	Anger	Indifference
More sensitive to	Own feelings	Not sensitive	Others' feelings
When threatened, tends to	Run	Fight	Make peace
Relations with spouse/partner	Clingy	Jealous	Secure
Expresses affection	With words	With gifts	With touch
When feeling hurt	Cries	Argues	Withdraws
Emotional trauma causes	Anxiety	Denial	Depression
Confidence level	Timid	Outwardly self-confident	Inner confidence
Emotional subtotal:	_____	_____	_____

Physical Profile

Category	VATA	PITTA	KAPHA
Amount of hair	Average	Thinning	Thick
Hair type	Dry	Normal	Oily
Hair color	Light brown, blonde	Red, auburn	Dark brown, black
Skin	Dry, rough, or both	Soft, normal to oily	Oily, moist, cool
Skin temperature	Cold hands/feet	Warm	Cool
Complexion	Darker	Pink-red	Pale-white
Eyes	Small	Medium	Large
Whites of eyes	Blue/brown	Yellow or red	Glossy white
Size of teeth	Very large or very small	Small–medium	Medium–large
Weight	Thin, hard to gain	Medium	Heavy, gains easily
Elimination	Dry, hard, thin, easily constipated	Many during day, soft to normal	Heavy, slow, thick, regular
Resting pulse			
Men	70–90	60–70	50–60
Women	80–100	70–80	60–70
Veins and tendons	Very prominent	Fairly prominent	Well covered
Physical subtotal:	_____	_____	_____

Fitness Profile

Category	VATA	PITTA	KAPHA
Exercise tolerance	Low	Medium	High
Endurance	Fair	Good	Excellent
Strength	Fair	Better than average	Excellent
Speed	Very good	Good	Not so fast
Competition	Doesn't like competitive pressure	Driven competitor	Deals easily with competitive pressure
Walking speed	Fast	Average	Slow and steady
Muscle tone	Lean, low body fat	Medium, with good definition	Brawny/bulky, with higher fat percentage
Runs like	Deer	Tiger	Bear
Body size	Small frame, lean or long	Medium frame	Large frame, fleshy
Reaction time	Quick	Average	Slow
Fitness subtotal:	_____	_____	_____

Totals

Your primary dosha is the column you scored highest in.

Profile	VATA	PITTA	KAPHA
Mental			
Behavioral			
Emotional			
Physical			
Fitness			
TOTAL:			

You Are a Vata

When in balance, you are bright, enthusiastic, creative, full of new ideas and initiative, idealistic and a visionary. You think fast, talk fast, love being with other people and enjoy travel and change. You are good at initiating things, but not necessarily at following them through. A clue to your constitution is to ask how many projects you have started or how many unfinished books you have on the bedside table at any one time. You are also prone to poor memory, lack of concentration, disorganization, fear and anxiety. You can suffer from nervous problems such as disorientation, panic attacks and mood swings.

You are so enthusiastic and full of energy that it's hard to keep you grounded. Much like the wind, you're changeable. Wonderfully creative with an artistic bent, you are sometimes accused of drumming to a different beat. You are unique and quite like it that way. You are very active, often restless and sometimes you find it hard to relax. You have a strong and sensitive spirit. You can be all these things. Just as the wind in balance provides movement and expression to the natural world, the balanced you is active, creative and gifted with a natural ability to express and communicate. When the wind in a Vata type rages like a hurricane, negative qualities quickly overshadow these positive attributes.

How do you know you have pushed your limits?

Signs and Symptoms of a Vata Imbalance

- Aching pain in the bones, cracking joints, arthritis and low backache
- Nervousness, anxiety, panic and fear
- Fatigue, lowered resistance to infection and weight loss
- Tinnitus, tingling and numbness
- Twitches, tics, tremors and spasms
- Dry skin and hair, brittle nails and chapped skin
- Constipation, gas, bloating, dry and hard stools and explosive diarrhea (aggravated by anxiety)
- Dislike of cold and wind
- Pain (cutting or migrating) and poor coordination
- Insomnia, restless sleep, tension and anxiety
- Insecurity, mental agitation, depression and restlessness
- Difficulty tolerating loud noises
- Spacey, scattered feeling
- Excess thinking or worrying

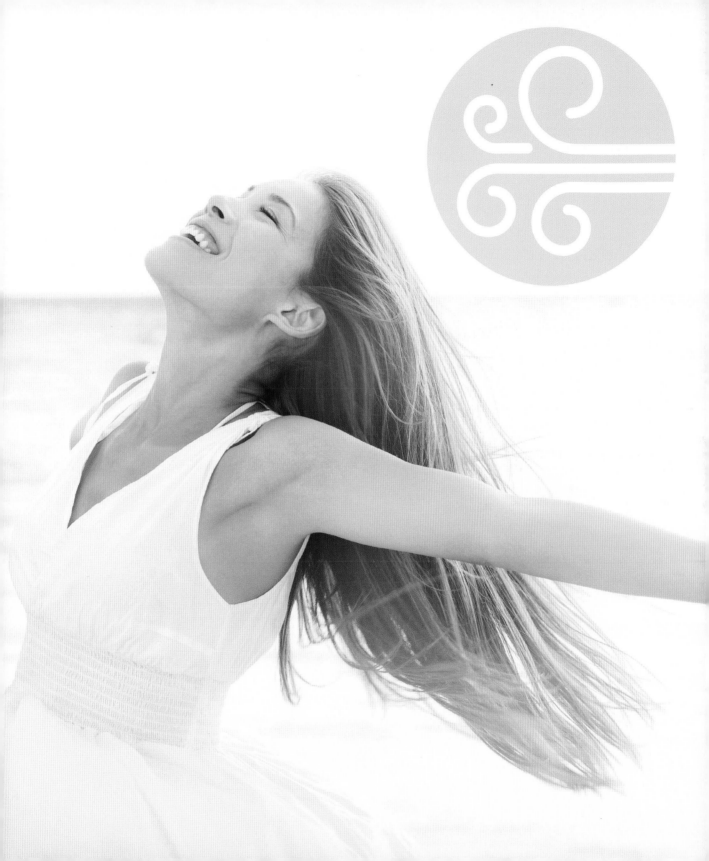

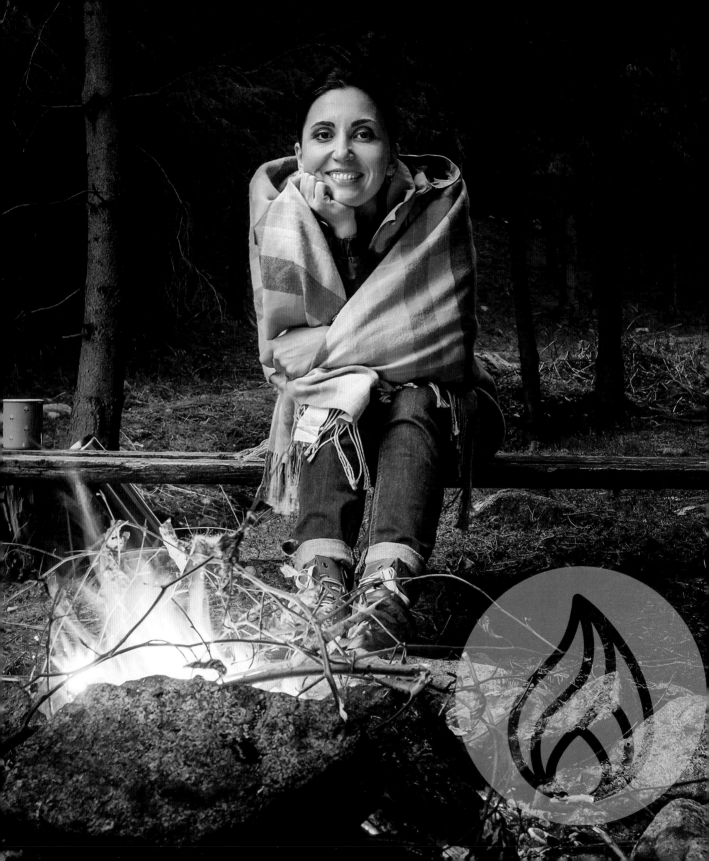

You Are a Pitta

You are extroverted and love to be the focus of attention. You enjoy competitive sports and games, either as a spectator or a participant. You are naturally brilliant—even fiery—and have good insight and a keen sense of discrimination. You tend to be highly focused, competitive, capable, courageous, energetic and are a clear communicator who gets right to the point. You like to solve problems—everybody's problems!

You generally have a good appetite and love to eat. In fact, you hate to miss a meal, and, when hungry, you can be irritable and prone to hypoglycemia, with headaches, dizziness, weakness and shaking. Your digestion is good, but when you get hot, agitated or angry, or eat too many hot, spicy or fried foods, you may suffer from indigestion, heartburn and loose, burning stools.

You are extremely methodical and organized. You can be rather obsessive about time, and I am sure that at some time or other, you've been called a perfectionist! In fact, you do not suffer fools easily.

You handle money prudently and are decisive, aggressive, ambitious and determined, often finding yourself in a position of leadership. Self-confidence and an entrepreneurial spirit are hallmarks of the balanced you.

Although you can usually control your emotions, under stress you can become irritable, angry and judgmental. You can also become overly intense, overly critical and too achievement oriented. There is a tendency to be a workaholic. You make a great friend but a feared enemy. Emotionally, you are quick to the heated emotions of anger, resentment and jealousy. You are also prone to inflammation, heartburn, acidity, diarrhea and migraines—it's important for you to just cool down.

Signs and Symptoms of a Pitta Imbalance

- Heat in the body
- Inflammation, often starting in the stomach and intestines, causing heartburn, acidity, gastritis and ulcers
- Inflammatory skin problems, such as eczema, urticaria, herpes and boils
- Blood disorders, anemia and high blood pressure
- Eye problems such as conjunctivitis, styes and blepharitis (inflammation of the eyelids)
- Hormonal problems, PMS and hot flashes
- Thirst, increased appetite, hypoglycemia, dizziness and diarrhea
- Anger, irritability, intolerance, aggression and arrogance
- Frustration, perfectionism, obsessions, addictions and insomnia between 10:00 p.m. and 2:00 a.m.
- Headaches and migraines

You Are a Kapha

You are grounded, stable and calm in thought, speech and action. You are easygoing and supportive in relationships. There is an element of steadiness to your step, a quality of serenity in your smile. Loyalty is your second name. You are physically strong and resilient. You are also placid, kind and thoughtful. You are sweet-natured, loyal and affectionate, and you hate confrontation.

You do not like change or the unpredictable aspects of life. You may have a tendency to be lazy—a couch potato who likes nothing better than to sit around, relax and do very little. Exertion does not come naturally to you, although vigorous exercise does make you feel really good.

People with more Kapha in their constitutions tend to be of larger proportions, with a robust frame and padded joints; thick, smooth skin that may tend toward oiliness; and rich, wavy hair. Your appetite is stable, although you are often not very hungry first thing in the morning, when you tend to feel sleepy. You love food and tend to comfort eat. Your digestion is slow and sluggish, as is your metabolism, which means weight gain is something you often battle with.

Factors that can cause your dosha to increase include a diet that contains too many deep-fried, sweet or heavy foods; overconsumption of ice-cold foods or beverages; exposure to cold and damp; daytime sleep and lack of exercise.

Signs and Symptoms of a Kapha Imbalance

- Feeling slow, heavy, lethargic, foggy-minded and unmotivated
- Mucus buildup, bronchial congestion, hay fever and asthma
- Weight gain, slow metabolism, excess salivation, nausea and heaviness after eating
- Metabolic syndrome and type 2 diabetes
- Fluid retention and lymphatic congestion
- General lethargy
- Poor circulation
- Possessiveness, greed, stubbornness and aversion to change
- Low thyroid function and high cholesterol
- Depression

But I Am a Combination of Doshas—What Do I Do?

If you find that you are predominantly two doshas, then this is how it works in each season.

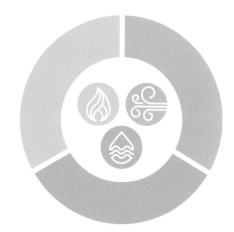

In summer (Pitta season):

- If you are Vata-Pitta, follow the Pitta recommendations.
- If you are Vata-Kapha, follow the Vata recommendations.
- If you are Pitta-Kapha, follow the Pitta recommendations.

In fall and early winter (Vata season):

- If you are Vata-Pitta, follow the Vata recommendations.
- If you are Vata-Kapha, follow the Vata recommendations.
- If you are Pitta-Kapha, follow the Pitta recommendations.

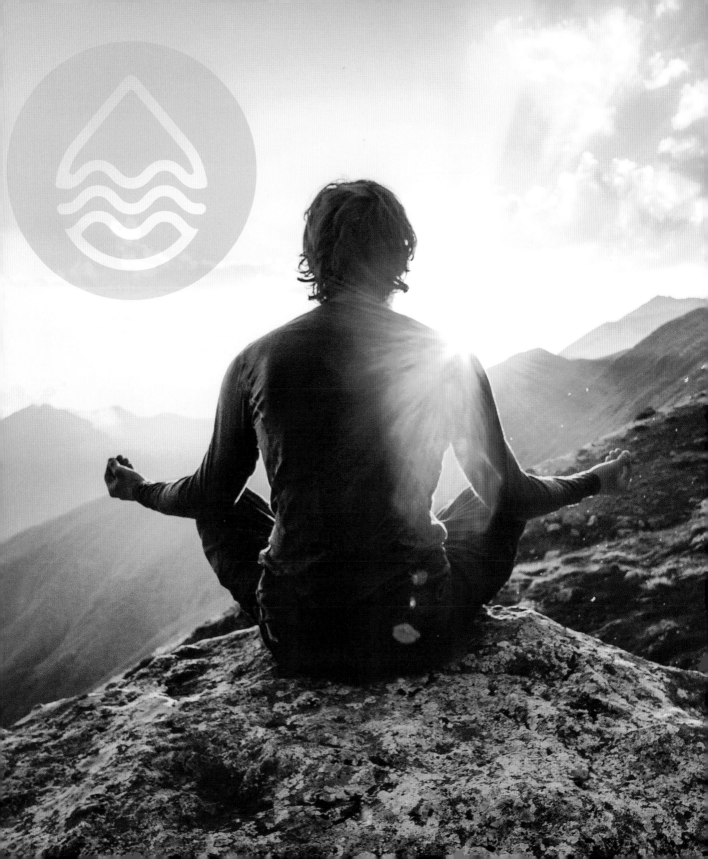

In late winter and spring (Kapha season):

- If you are Vata-Pitta, follow the Pitta recommendations.
- If you are Vata-Kapha, follow the Kapha recommendations.
- If you are Pitta-Kapha, follow the Kapha recommendations.

THE IMPORTANCE OF DIGESTION

Your dosha is important, and it's fun to see what metabolic type you are, but just as important is your state of agni. *Agni* (digestive fire) is literally the strength of your digestion, and in Western terms, we call it your metabolism. This is the process of changing your food into nutrients for your cells. However, your agni is more than just processing food into nutrients. It's also how you process your emotions and your sensory experiences. Your agni is essential for you to function effectively, and when your agni is functioning well, whatever you eat gets digested and absorbed by the body. You feel good and have lots of vitality. How do you know if your agni is functioning properly? Ask yourself if you are sleepy after a meal. If you find yourself longing for a nap by mid-afternoon, you probably have low agni.

What happens if your agni is low? What you cannot digest turns into digestive toxins, or what is called ama.

GOT AMA (TOXINS)?

How do you know you have ama? Let's start with the colon. Do you have regular, daily bowel movements with well-formed stools? This is a healthy colon. Or do your stools tend to sink? Do they have a particularly bad odor? Any signs of poor digestion such as gas, bloating, constipation, burping, heartburn or loose stools? These are all direct signs of ama buildup. But hang on! What is so wrong with ama?

Ama means "toxins" and there are two types: water-based toxins and fat-based toxins. Water-based toxins get easily flushed through the system due to our normal ability to detoxify, but fat-based toxins can accumulate. When our digestive system is not functioning well due to our diet and lifestyle, we build up these fat-based toxins. It is the fat-based toxins that we call ama and that create weight gain, sluggishness, foggy thinking, digestive issues, skin rashes, allergies and fatigue. Eventually, if we don't eliminate these fat-based toxins, the body becomes inflamed. It is inflammation that creates disease. Ama needs to be fully addressed before you can feel good again.

Do you have ama? Take this short questionnaire to determine your levels of ama.

Ama Questionnaire

For each question, rate your matching characteristics on a scale from 0 to 5:

0–1 doesn't apply, 2–3 sometimes applies, 4–5 strongly applies

- I often feel a sense of blockage in my body (such as constipation or congestion).
- I often have difficulty digesting food.
- I feel foggy when I wake up in the morning.
- I tend to feel weak for no apparent reason.
- I often feel lethargic and unmotivated.
- I feel the need to cough regularly.
- I become easily exhausted, both mentally and physically.
- I frequently feel depressed.
- I often have no taste for food.
- I catch a cold several times a year.

Add up your total score. A score of 0–19 indicates a low level of ama; 20–34 indicates a moderate amount of ama; 35–50 indicates a high amount of ama.

LET'S GET STARTED: TIPS FOR SUCCESS

TIP #1: Keep it simple. There are no complicated formulas to work out trying to find the right ratios of carbohydrates, proteins, fats and sugars. There are no calories to count and no foods to weigh. I don't even want you to weigh yourself. In fact, throw away the scale!

TIP #2: Do not think of this as a diet. Diets don't work. Here are the two main reasons your diets likely have not worked in the past:

- Diets actually slow weight loss. That's because the stress of dieting produces two hormones: adrenaline and cortisol. These hormones are considered a trigger for survival, and our body slows the rate of weight loss to concentrate on the perceived threat to survival. That threat to survival is your reduced calorie intake! Your body is doing what it is designed to do, and that's keep you alive.

- Diets don't actually cause us to change. We can all change our eating habits for a few weeks. In fact, we can do anything for a short period of time, as evidenced by the large amount of "change your life/health/relationship/finances in thirty days" books. After about thirty days, we start feeling deprived and begin slipping back into old habits. Even the Ayurveda cleanse is only the first step in your ultimate journey to health.

TIP #3: Create a stress-free rhythm. Here's how:

- Take a look at your schedule and eliminate any nonessential commitments while doing the cleanse.

- Allow time for yourself and for your body to rest and rejuvenate.

- Practice dynamic and restorative yoga regularly throughout the cleanse. It is ideal to practice with a teacher who knows you, but if that's not an option, I have created a sequence of restorative poses to help you. If you would like to join me with your yoga or meditation, go to www.theholistichighway.com/bookspecial and type in the password "Ayurveda." Here you'll find videos and audio to accompany the book, and we can do this together.

TIP #4: Eliminate caffeine, tobacco, recreational drugs and alcohol. It is best to try and limit the number of caffeinated beverages you drink. If you are used to drinking your morning coffee and find that you have a strong reaction to eliminating it completely, such as feeling ill or getting a headache, then it is best to taper off slowly. The same is true for tobacco products or any recreational drugs you may be using. Avoid alcohol completely throughout the cleanse.

TIP #5: Get plenty of rest. Have a regular sleep routine. This means going to bed and getting up at the same time each day. Aim for going to bed about 10:00 p.m. and start waking up around sunrise. Turn off electronics at least one hour before bed. The blue light from all electronics—and yes, that includes your phone—will stimulate your sleep-wake cycle.

TIP #6: Cleansing is not just a physical process. This cleanse is not just a physical cleanse but also a mental and emotional one. I want you to handle emotional stress through some simple suggestions. I will be giving you some journal topics as you go through the cleanse.

TIP #7: Stock your Ayurveda kitchen and medicine cabinet. Even if you haven't figured out your dosha yet, there are a few basic principles that will be true for any Ayurvedic pantry.

- Just say NO to processed foods. Okay, let's get a big garbage bag, because we are going to toss out all those ama-producing processed foods and create space in your pantry for delicious whole foods and spices that will have you feeling wonderful. So, toss out the sugared cereal and any other products containing sugar so you can start feeling better from the inside out. Yes, even those protein bars are processed—ditch them too! (I often have clients ask me, "What about my spouse and kids? Will they like these foods?" And I answer by asking, "Well, do you love your family? Do they really need those cocoa puffs, goldfish snacks or chocolate chip cookies?" I didn't think so. This cleanse will benefit the whole family.)

- Go through your fridge too. It doesn't have to happen all at once, but start slowly on your path away from toxic fruits and veggies that have been doused with pesticides and insecticides and are ultimately devoid of their vitamins, minerals and flavor.

- Stock your kitchen with nutritious life-giving foods. Before you take a trip to the grocery store, all prepared to load up with healthy foods, slow down. As tempting as it may be to rush off and fill your grocery bags with organic fruits and veggies, I don't want you spending a small fortune on your new foods without a clue about what to do with them. I'm going to break it down for you so that we are all on the same page. Choose fresh fruits, veggies, grains and whole foods. We will be adding some essential herbal supplements designed to increase your agni as well as some massage oils and other self-care essentials.

SUGAR CRAVINGS: "But, Kerry, there's no way I can get through the day without something sweet!" I hear this all the time. Let's look at why you may be craving something sweet. First, did you eat enough at your last meal to see you through to the next? Second, what is going on in your life right now? You may be looking to self-medicate and calm your nervous system. Don't worry, the sweet taste is included in plenty of foods on this cleanse. I bet you didn't know that rice, oatmeal, the nut milks and most of your veggies are sweet! Just like any habit, it is difficult at first but then gets better. By the time you have gone through the pre-cleanse, you will not be craving processed sugars—I promise you!

TIP #8: You just gotta jump in and start cooking. Before you whip out your ol' apron or start sharpening the knives, remember that cooking is a wonderful self-care practice that you can do not just for yourself but for your family and friends too.

- I get it! Maybe cooking has never been your thing. Believe me—I really get it. It was never my thing either. My idea of a gourmet meal was to buy a precooked chicken, a bag of salad and a bottle of Greek dressing. Add a bottle of wine, and I thought I was nourishing my body. However, fast-forward several years and I now write meal plans that are dosha-specific, and I have written this book full of tried-and-tested recipes. Each meal plan and recipe has been developed based upon the nourishing qualities of the ingredients. There is something very empowering about preparing, cooking and nourishing your body and mind. Enjoy that feeling!

- As you cook these meals, explore the tastes and textures. I love the smell of the spices as they cook and the sizzle of the seeds. How about you? I play music while I cook and sing along to my heart's content. I have even been known to bop around the house with my wooden spoon, much to the amusement of my family. In other words—have fun with it.

TIP #9: Use your health tracker. The health tracker (page 209) is your tool to gauge how you feel and how much you are improving. If something causes a reaction, like certain foods, herbs or oils, then you can easily identify the problem through the health tracker. How will you know you feel better, look better, sleep better and move better if you are not tracking it? So, I also suggest that you take before and after photos, as well as photos throughout the cleanse. You'll notice that your skin will start to glow, your hair will become glossier and your eyes will shine. (I know, it makes you sound like a golden retriever.) You will get used to your gradual change over the 25 days. These photos will be clear indicators of how you change during the cleanse.

TIP #10: Timing is everything, so follow your internal clock. The Ayurveda cleanse will encourage you to follow nature's clock or daily routine. There are certain times of the day that are better to exercise, to eat certain foods, to meditate, to do your spiritual practice, to work . . . even to eliminate! The Ayurveda daily clock is based upon doshas, which govern certain hours in the day. See how matching your mealtimes, sleep cycle and activities to these cycles makes a huge difference in your health.

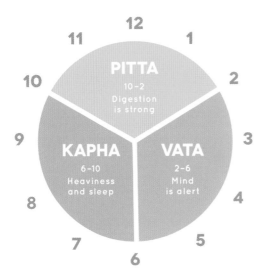

- **6:00 a.m.–10:00 a.m. Kapha time.** This is the time that Kapha increases, which means a slow and steady energy. This is the best time for exercise and physical labor, as Kapha is heavy and supports greater physical strength. Eat lightly at this time, as your agni is not strong. Ever slept late and woken up at 9:00 a.m.? How did you feel? Did you feel sluggish and a little heavy after sleeping in? This is because you have woken up in Kapha time, when the energy is heavy.

- **10:00 a.m.–2:00 p.m. Pitta time.** This is the time that Pitta increases. This is the best time of day to eat your biggest meal, as your digestive fire is the strongest in the middle of the day. It is also the best time to be productive. The Pitta tendency to organize, manage and solve problems will be strong, so go with it and plan accordingly.

- **2:00 p.m.–6:00 p.m. Vata time.** This is the best time for mental and creative energy, as the nervous system is more active. We may even feel a little more scattered and unfocused. The Vata energy will want us moving—so not a good time for a strategy meeting. However, it is the perfect time to be creative. Think outside the box, write that blog, draw that picture and paint that scene. Do you know that craving sweets at this time indicates exhaustion, blood-sugar issues, poor digestion or not enough nutrition at lunch to get you through your day?

- **6:00 p.m.–10:00 p.m. Kapha time.** Kapha starts increasing as we head into the evening hours. This is the best time to begin settling down for sleep and to relax. Kapha is heavy, and with cortisol levels dropping at this time . . . you should be getting sleepy! Have a light dinner, as your digestive fire has slowed as well, and you will not digest your food well at night. This is not the time to bring work home or start a project. Nurture yourself by using this time to relax.

- **10:00 p.m.–2:00 a.m. Pitta time.** Pitta increases again, and you should be sleeping. The liver (Pitta organ) engages in detoxifying and rejuvenating at this time. Have you ever stayed up late and felt like you got a second wind? Have you ever said that you do your best work in the wee hours of the morning? That's because the Pitta energy has kicked back in again. Instead of using that energy to rejuvenate, which is what happens when we are sleeping, if you are constantly up and awake during this time, the natural detoxing and rejuvenation that should be taking place is disturbed. (Did you know that staying up past 10:00 p.m. is a common cause of slow metabolism and weight gain?)

- **2:00 a.m.–6:00 a.m. Vata time.** The energy of Vata kicks back in again and the central nervous system starts stirring just before the sun rises. This is the best time to naturally wake up—just before sunrise. There is movement in the colon, and this is the best time to eliminate. This is also an especially good time for any kind of spiritual practice, and it is the perfect time to exercise, as the body naturally wants to move. Do you tend to wake up around 2:00 a.m. and have trouble getting back to sleep? This indicates that there is a Vata imbalance in your system.

What's great about this cleanse is that it is tailored to you; you will be cleansing in a way that is right for your body. It will give you increased energy, more focus and an overall sense of well-being. So, now you have everything you need. Let's get started with the pre-cleanse.

NOTE: Each recipe in the following chapters is written for a Vata dosha, but with clear instructions on how you can modify for Pittas and Kaphas too.

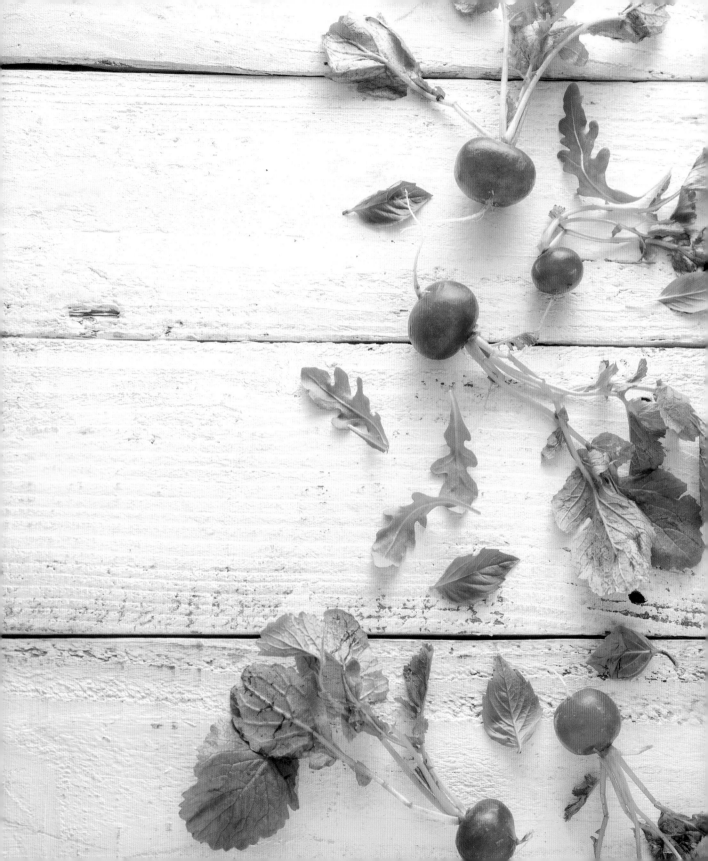

Chapter 2

PHASE 1
DAYS 1 TO 11

"All disease starts in the gut." —Hippocrates

PRE-CLEANSE: REVAMP YOUR HABITS

This phase is all about cleaning up your diet and lifestyle to prepare for the active cleanse in phase 2. We start by revamping your habits in order to improve your gut health. You will use foods such as beets and apples to scrub away the toxins and promote good gut health. As you reduce your intake of fast foods, processed foods, meat, refined sugars and sweets, you'll focus on eating as many simple whole foods as possible. This will set the stage for a more productive cleanse and will help your body ease into detox mode.

Just remember that it's easy to be overwhelmed when trying something new. I am going to make this as easy as possible for you, but there will be days when you make mistakes—none of us is perfect! However, stay the course. The results will be well worth it, I promise. But, go at the pace that is right for you, and remember that this is the start of a lifestyle shift that will keep you in optimal health over your whole, much longer, life.

DAILY ROUTINE

I have provided a daily dosha routine that will most benefit you on the cleanse. As you follow your daily routine, take a look at the day-by-day suggestions for your pre-cleanse during days 1 to 11.

Days 1 to 8 of the pre-cleanse prepare you by eliminating trigger foods that are clogging, heavy and acidic. This is preparing your body to shift to a more alkaline state and get ready for the active cleanse. Days 9 to 11 of the pre-cleanse involve *internal oleation*—the ingestion of ghee. If you are vegan, you can use sesame oil instead. This will serve to loosen the sticky, fat-soluble toxins and help them move toward the digestive tract.

Once the oiling loosens the ama (toxins), the ingestion of castor oil flushes it from the body. This is a onetime purgative procedure produced by the qualities of the castor oil on the evening of day eleven. This will not remove all the toxins from the body but will help clean out the toxins that weaken your agni (digestive fire). Once this is done, your agni will more efficiently handle the next active phase of the cleanse. During these three oleation days, eat normal dosha foods: apples, Beet Slaw (page 39) and Energizing Potassium Tonic (page 40). In other words, maintain all the good practices you have put in place and follow your daily routines.

Phase 1 Daily Routine

	VATA	PITTA	KAPHA
Wake Up	½ hour before sunrise (in spring and summer in the Northern Hemisphere, feel free to get up just before sunrise)	1 hour before sunrise (in spring and summer in the Northern Hemisphere, feel free to get up ½ hour before sunrise)	1½ hours before sunrise (in spring and summer in the Northern Hemisphere, feel free get up 45 minutes before sunrise)
Drink	Warm water with lemon juice and raw honey or Vata Cleansing Tea (page 31)	¼ cup (60 ml) aloe vera juice or Pitta Cooling Tea (page 31)	Warm ginger tea or Kapha Stimulating Tea (page 31)
Nose	Add a few drops of sesame oil or nasya oil into both nostrils (see page 35).		
Exercise	Follow yoga gentle stretching (see page 108).		
Shower	Massage with sesame oil before taking a hot shower or bath.	Massage with coconut oil before taking a warm shower or bath.	Massage with mustard oil before taking a hot shower or bath.
Facial Serum	Vata Facial Serum (page 33)	Pitta Facial Serum (page 33)	Kapha Facial Serum (page 33)
Meditation Practice	Spend 15 minutes minimum in your daily spiritual practice. See journal suggestions.		
Breakfast	Cooked breakfast (pages 43–61). Follow with 1 raw green apple.	Cooked breakfast (pages 43–61). Follow with 1 raw green apple.	Cooked breakfast (pages 43–61). Follow with 1 raw green apple.
Mid-Morning	Take 2 trikatu tablets (see page 37). Eat an apple (if hungry). Vata Cleansing Tea (page 31)	Eat an apple (if hungry). Pitta Cooling Tea (page 31)	Take 2 trikatu tablets (see page 37). Eat an apple (if hungry). Kapha Stimulating Tea (page 31)
Lunch (12 p.m. to 2 p.m.)	Follow a balancing meal for your dosha. Add Beet Slaw (page 39). Add Energizing Potassium Tonic (page 40) at lunch or dinner. Follow with 1 green apple. Take a few minutes to rest after your meal.	Follow a balancing meal for your dosha. Add Beet Slaw (page 39). Add Energizing Potassium Tonic (page 40) at lunch or dinner. Follow with 1 green apple. Take a few minutes to walk after your meal.	Take 2 trikatu tablets (see page 37). Follow a balancing meal for your dosha. Add Beet Slaw (page 39). Add Energizing Potassium Tonic (page 40) (optional). Follow with 1 green apple. Take a brisk walk after your meal.

	VATA	PITTA	KAPHA
Mid-Afternoon	Vata Cleansing Tea (page 31)	Pitta Cooling Tea (page 31)	Kapha Stimulating Tea (page 31)
Dinner (5:30 p.m. to 7:30 p.m.)	Follow a balancing meal for your dosha. Add Energizing Potassium Tonic (page 40). Follow with 1 green apple. Take a few minutes to rest after your meal.	Follow a balancing meal for your dosha. Add Energizing Potassium Tonic (page 40). Follow with 1 green apple. Take a few minutes to walk after your meal.	Follow a balancing meal for your dosha. Add Energizing Potassium Tonic (page 40). Follow with 1 green apple. Take a brisk walk after your meal.
Sunset	Do gentle stretching or take a rejuvenating walk.	Take a walk.	Take a brisk walk.
Journal Practice	See journal suggestions.		
Nighttime	Take 2 triphala tablets or 1 tsp triphala powder in warm water (see page 37).	Take 2 triphala tablets or 1 tsp triphala powder in warm water (see page 37).	Take 2 triphala tablets or 1 tsp triphala powder in warm water (see page 37).
Massage	Massage soles of feet with sesame oil.	Massage soles of feet with sunflower or coconut oil.	Massage soles of feet with sesame or mustard oil.
Essential Oil	Add 1 drop lavender to pillow for restful sleep.	Add 1 drop sandalwood for cooling and revitalizing sleep.	Add 1 drop bergamot for refreshing sleep.
Mantra Before Sleep	Let go of worries and conflicts of the day.	Let go of what I can't control.	Let go of what does not serve me anymore.

DAY 1

Start your day by following the routine that is right for your dosha. Follow this routine for the rest of your pre-cleanse; however, on Day 1 you will also eliminate all dairy (except ghee). Start your triphala and trikatu (see page 37). Take the triphala at night before bed and the trikatu in mid-morning and mid-afternoon. Eat the foods that are right for your dosha, but remember that the recipes are just suggestions; feel free to eat any whole grains, fruits and vegetables that feel right for you.

Journal Entry: You are not alone. Who do you have a connection with? Who is your biggest cheerleader? How do they let you know they are there for you?

DAY 2

Eliminate alcohol and sodas.

Journal Entry: Some of the things that make me happy are . . .

DAY 3

Eliminate all sugars—that is, anything that has added sugar in it. Fruit is still okay.

Journal Entry: My saddest memory is . . .

DAY 4

Eliminate all animal products. (Don't forget that eggs and yogurt are animal products.)

Journal Entry: I deal with anger and frustration by . . .

DAY 5

Eliminate coffee and all processed foods. Now if the thought of going without your morning cup of joe has you in a panic, don't worry. Simply reduce your coffee consumption by half. That means you can add more water to your cup or just drink a little less coffee. Caffeine is a stimulant that wears out the adrenal glands, resulting in fatigue. It's going to be hard to be full of vitality and health if you are downing a pot of coffee every day.

Journal Entry: How easy is it for you to forgive those who have caused you pain?

DAY 6

Eliminate all caffeine, including chocolate.

Journal Entry: Observe yourself. What do you love most about yourself? Can you thank your body for being strong enough to bring you to where you are today?

DAY 7

Eliminate fruit juices and dried fruit.

Journal Entry: What is the dominant emotion in your life right now?

DAY 8

Eliminate fresh fruit and nuts.

Journal Entry: Take time to write about your thoughts, feelings and concerns during the cleanse so far. Are you feeling positive or negative?

DAY 9

Start internal oleation: Between 6:00 a.m. and 7:00 a.m. take 1 tablespoon (15 ml) of ghee or sesame oil in 1 cup (240 ml) of hot water. Take the ghee or oil in liquid form on an empty stomach. About ½ hour later, have another glass of warm water. If you feel slightly nauseated, try some fresh lemon juice in your warm water.

Journal Entry: My favorite weekend ritual is . . .

DAY 10

Between 6:00 a.m. and 7:00 a.m., take 2 tablespoons (30 ml) of ghee or sesame oil in 1 cup (240 ml) of hot water. Take the oil or ghee in liquid form on an empty stomach. About ½ hour later, have another glass of warm water. If you feel slightly nauseated, try some fresh lemon juice in your warm water.

Journal Entry: The holiday traditions I most look forward to are . . .

DAY 11

Morning: Between 6:00 a.m. and 7:00 a.m., take 3 tablespoons (45 ml) of ghee or sesame oil in 1 cup (240 ml) of hot water. Take the oil or ghee in liquid form on an empty stomach. About ½ hour later, have another glass of warm water. If you feel slightly nauseated, try some fresh lemon juice in your warm water.

Journal Entry: Things I always did with my dad when I was small were . . .

Evening: Have a very light meal. Before bedtime, enjoy a 15- to 20-minute hot bath or shower. Then take 2 tablespoons (30 ml) of castor oil. You can take it straight or put the castor oil in ½ cup (120 ml) of warm water. The laxative effects will normally occur between 4 to 6 hours after ingesting. Expect to be awakened in the early morning with a gentle but urgent need to eliminate.

Journal Entry: If you could only take three items with you in a hurry from your home, what would they be? Why did you choose what you did?

IMPORTANT AYURVEDA PRACTICES

Cleansing Teas

Sipping warm teas throughout the day is a highly effective way to flush out ama and other toxins from the body. What follows are basic detoxifying teas for each dosha. Simply place the ingredients in a medium saucepan with 4 cups (960 ml) of filtered water, bring the water to a boil for 5 minutes and then steep for 2 to 5 minutes. Always add the lemon while the tea is steeping. Strain the tea into a teapot or thermos before enjoying.

Vata Cleansing Tea

1 tsp cumin seeds

½ tsp coriander seeds

1 tsp fennel seeds

½ tsp freshly grated ginger

Lemon juice, as desired

Raw organic sugar, such as Sucanat (optional)

Pitta Cooling Tea

1 tsp fennel seeds

1 tsp coriander seeds

½ tsp cumin seeds

10 fresh mint leaves

Lemon juice, as desired

Raw organic sugar, such as Sucanat (optional)

Kapha Stimulating Tea

1 tsp cumin seeds

½ tsp coriander seeds

1 cinnamon or licorice stick

10 fresh basil leaves

Lemon juice, as desired

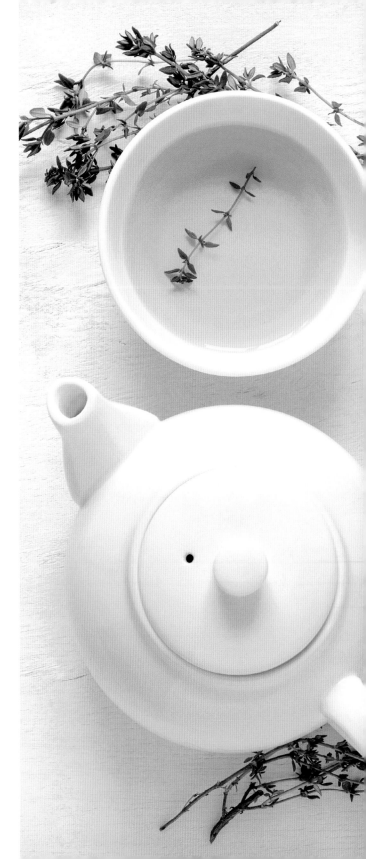

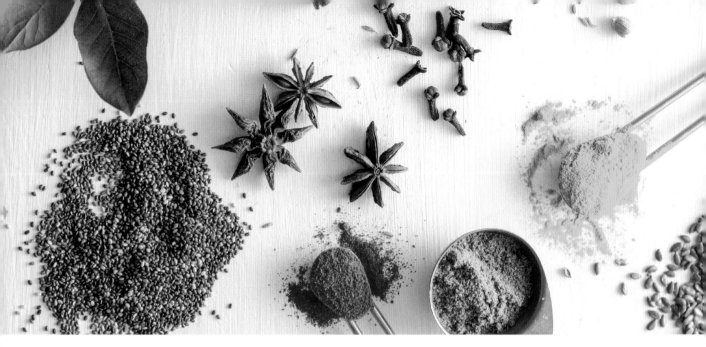

Spice It Up!

Spices are an important part of cleansing. We can use food as medicine to improve digestion as well as reduce ama and inflammation. These are the cleansing spices that you will be using in the following recipes when asked to add your dosha spice mix. These spices are what makes the cleanse unique for you.

For the following dosha-specific spice mixes, place all the ingredients in an electric grinder or spice mill and grind them. Pour the mixture into a bowl and stir with a spoon until they're well combined. Transfer it to an airtight container and store at cool room temperature. I recommend using these mixtures within 1 month for the best potency.

Vata Spice Mix

1 tbsp (9 g) coriander seeds

1 tbsp (9 g) cumin seeds

1 tbsp (9 g) ground turmeric

1 tbsp (9 g) dried basil

2 tsp (6 g) powdered ginger

2 tsp (10 g) salt

1 tsp asafetida (hing)

Pitta Spice Mix

2 tbsp (18 g) coriander seeds

2 tbsp (18 g) fennel seeds

2 tbsp (18 g) cumin seeds

2 tbsp (6 g) chopped mint leaves

1 tbsp (9 g) whole cardamom seeds

1 tbsp (9 g) ground turmeric

Kapha Spice Mix

1 tbsp (9 g) coriander seeds

1 tbsp (9 g) cumin seeds

1 tbsp (9 g) fennel seeds

1 tbsp (9 g) mustard seeds

1 tbsp (9 g) fenugreek seeds

1 tbsp (9 g) cardamom seeds

1 tbsp (9 g) poppy seeds

1 tbsp (9 g) ground cinnamon

1 tbsp (9 g) ground ginger

Facial Serums

Whether you already have fantastic skin or are suffering from problematic skin, the sheer variety of serums can be overwhelming. To ensure you have one that is right for your skin, pick the serum for your dosha. Apply to a damp face after you have used your facial wash and your skin will start glowing!

Vata Facial Serum

2 tbsp (30 ml) jojoba oil

¼ cup (60 ml) almond oil

3-4 drops rose or geranium essential oil

Pitta Facial Serum

2 tbsp (30 ml) almond oil

¼ cup (60 ml) sunflower oil

5-6 drops sandalwood or rose oil

Kapha Facial Serum

2 tbsp (30 ml) flaxseed oil

¼ cup (60 ml) almond oil

3-4 drops lavender or rosemary oil

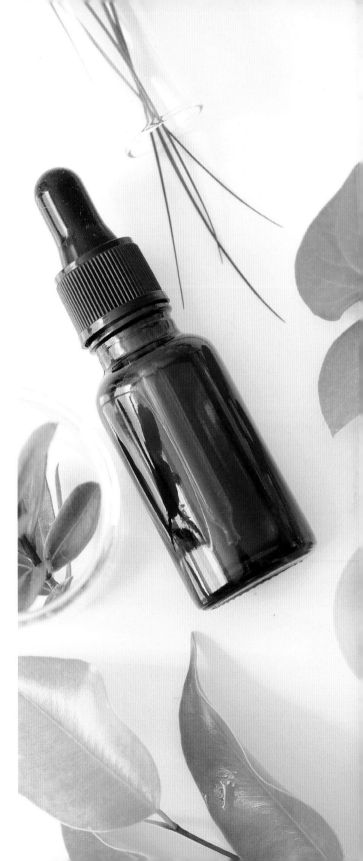

Scrape Your Tongue

Tongue scraping is a method of cleaning the tongue to remove any coating, mucous and other debris that may have accumulated overnight. This is most easily achieved using a well-designed tongue scraper commonly made from stainless steel, silver or copper. If you are not scraping your tongue in the mornings, please read on.

Do you have bad morning breath or a white-colored coating on your tongue? If you haven't checked, have a look in the mirror and you will probably notice this.

While brushing and flossing remove bacteria from the teeth and gums, it is the forgotten bacteria living on our tongues that can cause bad breath and even interfere with our sense of taste. Nearly 50 percent of our oral bacteria live in the deep crevices of the tongue and are a major source of bad breath, gum disease and tooth decay. The coating provides a base for the microbes to grow on; removing the coating is vital to killing bacteria.

This toxic residue comes from all over the body. During sleep when the body is resting, the digestive system works to detoxify itself. These toxins (ama) are deposited on the surface of the tongue via the internal excretory channels and are responsible for the coating usually seen on the tongue first thing in the morning. The coating may be yellow, white, black or bluish in color. Up to 40 percent of toxins from the day before will come up on your tongue the following day, brought in from the respiratory, digestive and nervous systems.

Here's how to scrape your tongue:

1. Get the right tongue scraper! Dental research has found that using a tongue scraper is many times more effective at removing bacteria from the tongue than a toothbrush. The sweeping action of a tongue scraper will collect the waste deposits in its U-bend, allowing the bacteria to be rinsed away under the tap.

2. Brush and floss your teeth. This needs to be done first as some toxins from your teeth and gums will fall onto your tongue.

3. Hold the tongue scraper gently in both hands. Open your mouth and place the curved part as far back on the tongue as is comfortable without gagging.

4. Gently pull the scraper forward over the surface of the tongue. Do this a few times.

5. When finished, thoroughly rinse the tongue scraper under running water and hang to dry.

6. This should ideally be done first thing in the morning as the body's metabolism will start working and the toxic residue will begin to reabsorb back into various organs and channels if tongue scraping is not done.

Daily tongue scraping also helps improve digestion by activating saliva production and stoking the agni (digestive fire) for the day ahead. A healthy tongue will look clean and be pinkish in color. With continued daily scraping, you will find your overall health improving.

Drink Plenty of Water

Dehydration is probably the most common cause of digestive problems, headaches, fatigue, lymph congestion and poor detoxification function. Thus, one of our first priorities during the cleanse is to deeply rehydrate all the cells of the body, especially the digestive tract. Sip plain, boiled, hot water every 10 to 15 minutes throughout the day. This will not only rehydrate but also dilate the lymphatic system, allowing lymph to flow easily. Do not use ice in your water.

Eat an Apple a Day to Keep the Doctor Away

Raw, sour apples are incredibly good for cleansing, so make apples part of your meal. The two ingredients in apples that pack a detoxifying punch are pectin and malic acid.

Pectin acts as a detoxifier of the gut wall and is used to regulate bowel movements. It can help firm up loose stools and reduce inflammation associated with diarrhea, as well as help with constipation. Pectin can be useful in treating diseases such as colitis, irritable bowel syndrome and other digestive disorders.

Malic acid dilates the bile ducts, which allows for more bile flow. Increased bile flow lowers the amount of cholesterol and fat in the liver. Malic acid is also an effective metal chelator, which means it's capable of binding to toxic metals, such as aluminum or lead that may have accumulated in the liver, and deactivating them. This considerably reduces the risk of toxicity. (Did you know that 80 percent of all gallstones are cholesterol stones? Malic acid softens and ultimately dissolves gallstones.) The more sour an apple, the more malic acid it contains. So, go ahead and look for the greenest apples. I find that Granny Smith apples are generally the most sour.

Use Nasya Oil

Nasya is the name of the practice of applying oils directly into the nostrils. This balances the sinuses, throat and head, resulting in an improved immune system, better circulation and mental clarity and focus. This means fewer sinus infections, less congestion and allergy and asthma relief. Here's how to do it:

- Place a drop of nasya or sesame oil on your ring finger and gently apply it into each nostril.
- Massage with a gentle circular motion inside each nostril.

It is not recommended to do nasya if you have a cold, a sinus infection or the flu.

PRE-CLEANSE MEAL PLAN

I have tried to keep the recipes simple for you by aligning them for Vata, as this is the first dosha to go out of balance. However, if you are Kapha or Pitta, I have included the adjustments at the bottom of each recipe so that you can adjust it for your dosha. If you find that you are predominantly two doshas, then use the adjustments listed on pages 20 and 22.

Shopping List

This list will help you stock up on the supplies you'll need for this phase of the cleanse. These are just the ingredients you need for the spices, teas and tonics. Depending upon which meals you choose, your shopping list may vary.

Remember, these meals are just suggestions; as long as you are eating healthy grains and organic vegetables, you can choose your own recipes. I find, though, that it is often easier to follow a menu, and that is why I have created the following meal plan for you.

Herbs and Products

- Triphala powder or tablets (all doshas; page 37)
- Trikatu tablets (Vatas and Kaphas only; page 37)
- Dosha teas (page 31)
- Oil for abhyanga (massage)
- Castor oil (internal grade)
- Nasya or sesame oil
- Tongue scraper

Groceries (buy organic as much as possible)

- 33 to 44 green apples
- 4–6 medium raw beets
- 1 bag rolled oats
- 1 box raisins
- Fruit (for Not Your Mother's Oatmeal, page 43)
- 1 bag raw spinach
- 1 bunch celery
- 11 medium zucchini
- 2 bunches raw parsley
- 1 bunch carrots
- 1 bag green beans

Spices and Garnishes

- Asafetida (hing)
- Black mustard seed
- Black and cayenne pepper
- Cilantro
- Cinnamon powder
- Coconut, unsweetened and shredded
- Coriander powder and whole seeds
- Cumin seed, whole
- Dijon mustard (optional)
- Fennel powder and whole seeds
- Gingerroot
- Mint, fresh or dried
- Nutmeg powder
- Turmeric powder

Sweeteners

- Barley malt
- Raw honey
- Turbinado sugar

Meal Plan for Pre-Cleanse

Feel free to mix and match the recipes to your liking.

	DAY 1	DAY 2	DAY 3	DAY 4	DAY 5
Breakfast	Dosha Tea (page 31) / Not Your Mother's Oatmeal (page 43)	Dosha Tea (page 31) / Veggie Breakfast Tacos and Salsa (page 44)	Dosha Tea (page 31) / Quinoa Bake with Warm Spiced Milk (page 47)	Dosha Tea (page 31) / Stewed Peaches with Dates, Cardamom and Almond Cream (page 48)	Dosha Tea (page 31) / Millet Cakes with Nut Butter (page 51)
Mid-Morning	Dosha Tea (page 31)	Mint Tea (page 62)	Ginger Tea (page 63)	Tulsi Tea (page 64)	Dandelion Tea (page 65)
Lunch	Braised Kale and Wild Rice Salad with Fennel (page 81)	Cleansing Buddha Bowl (page 70)	Chermoula and Pasta (page 82)	Quinoa Asparagus Pilaf (page 180)	Pumpkin Saffron Soup (page 85)
Mid-Afternoon	Agni-Boosting Tea (page 66)	Dosha Tea (page 31)	Breaktime Beneficial Broth (page 68)	Digestive Tea (page 67)	Saffron Lemonade (page 69)
Supper	Amazing Mushroom Soup (page 102)	Jicama Salad with Minty Tahini Sauce (page 94)	Black Bean Tacos with Mango Salsa (page 89)	Fenugreek and Dill Weight-Loss Soup (page 97)	Zucchini Noodles with Pesto (page 98)

	DAY 6	DAY 7	DAY 8	DAY 9	DAY 10	DAY 11
Breakfast	Dosha Tea (page 31) / Coconut Cucumber Smoothie (page 56)	Dosha Tea (page 31) / Yummy Breakfast Pancakes (page 55)	Dosha Tea (page 31) / Breakfast Rice (page 52)	Dosha Tea (page 31) / Stimulating Juice Cocktail (page 57)	Dosha Tea (page 31) / Upma (page 58)	Dosha Tea (page 31) / Detox Breakfast Stew (page 61)
Mid-Morning	Dosha Tea (page 31)	Mint Tea (page 62)	Ginger Tea (page 63)	Tulsi Tea (page 64)	Dandelion Tea (page 65)	Dosha Tea (page 31)
Lunch	Sumptuous Spinach Curry (page 73)	Easy Vegetable Stew (page 74)	Roasted Vegetable Bowl (page 78)	Anti-Inflammatory Broccoli Soup (page 77)	Cleansing Buddha Bowl (page 70)	One-Pot Shakshuka (page 86)
Mid-Afternoon	Agni-Boosting Tea (page 66)	Dosha Tea (page 31)	Breaktime Beneficial Broth (page 68)	Digestive Tea (page 67)	Saffron Lemonade (page 69)	Agni-Boosting Tea (page 66)
Supper	Cream of Asparagus Soup (page 166)	Pumpkin Pasta (page 106)	Saffron Lentil Risotto (page 105)	Winter Farro Salad (page 90)	Baked Tofu with Ginger Rice (page 93)	Cooling Coconut Curry Soup (page 101)

Take Triphala and Trikatu

In addition to the basic spices listed, there are two more herbs I want you to get: triphala and trikatu.

Triphala is a combination of three fruits and is known as a rejuvenating tonic that helps with digestion, detoxification and elimination. It is good for all three doshas and supports the respiratory, cardiovascular, urinary, reproductive and nervous systems. According to popular sources, it can reduce high blood pressure and improve liver function. It's been proven to be a powerful antioxidant, which means it protects cells from the damaging effects of free radicals. I want you to use triphala because it gently promotes internal cleansing and simultaneously works to improve digestion and nutrient absorption. Take two tablets at night before bed or 1 teaspoon of the powder in a glass of warm water.

Trikatu literally means "three pungents," or "three peppers." This herb is also used to support digestion, especially for Vatas and Kaphas. Because trikatu is so pungent, it clears excess mucus and congestion and has anti-inflammatory properties. Take this herb in between meals, about two hours after each meal for maximum effect. Take two tablets mid-morning and mid-afternoon.

PRE-CLEANSE RECIPES

Each of the following recipes were designed specifically for the pre-cleanse portion of your 25-day cleanse. Remember that the recipes are written for Vata with adaptations given for Pitta and Kapha.

Essential Detoxifying Recipes

The following two recipes are important parts of your meal plan during the pre-cleanse. Eat one or two servings of the beet slaw with your meals. Drink the tonic with lunch and/or dinner.

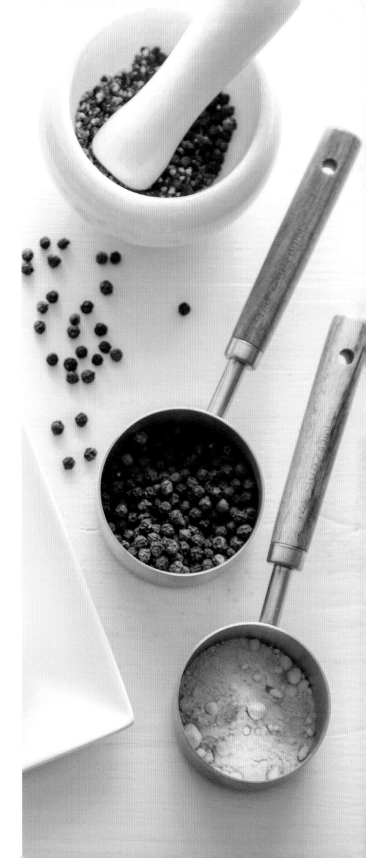

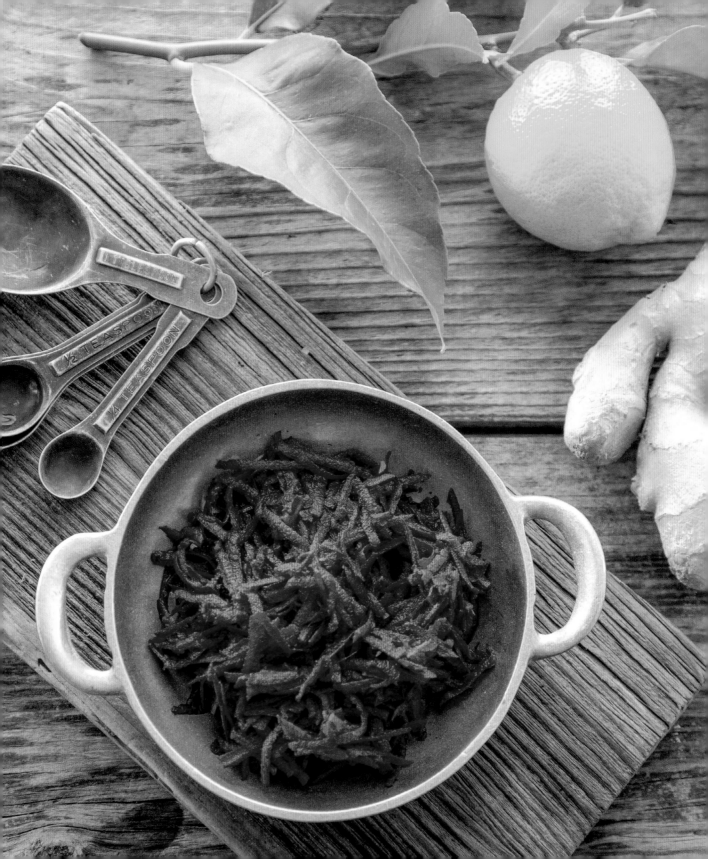

BEET SLAW

Your diet over the next 11 days will include more beets than you are perhaps used to. Beets are much more than a fall root vegetable. They are packed with antioxidants, vitamins and fiber. They also regulate cholesterol levels and bowel function. Beets are rich in beta-carotene and antioxidants, which make beets incredibly effective at cleansing the liver, particularly if you suffer from fatty liver disease. All this helps prevent the buildup of fats in this important detoxifying organ. Another benefit of beets is that they optimize the lymphatic system, further helping to remove toxins from the liver.

YIELD: 2 servings

1 medium raw beet, peeled and grated
Juice of ½ lemon
¼ tsp grated fresh ginger

Combine the beet, lemon juice and ginger in a bowl and serve as a side dish or topping. You can save this slaw for up to 24 hours in a sealed container in the refrigerator.

ENERGIZING POTASSIUM TONIC

This drink, which is surprisingly tasty and exceedingly high in potassium and electrolytes, is a nutritive drink during the pre-cleanse. It helps alleviate gas and bloating as well as heartburn. It is also an anti-inflammatory tonic, so it helps with joint pain, especially arthritis. Finally, as a detoxifying drink, it will help reduce any of those pesky cravings.

YIELD: 2 servings

4 cups (960 ml) water
5 raw carrots, chopped
2 celery ribs, chopped
1 raw zucchini, chopped
1½ cups (165 g) chopped green beans
1½ tsp (3 g) chopped fresh ginger
1 cup (30 g) chopped spinach
½ cup (30 g) chopped parsley

In a pot, bring the water to a boil. Place the carrots, celery, zucchini, green beans and ginger in the boiling water for approximately 8 minutes, keeping it at a low boil. Add the chopped spinach and parsley and cook for another 5 minutes, or until the vegetables are soft but not mushy.

Place them in a colander and drain, setting aside some of the veggie water. Process them in a blender until smooth. Add some of the reserved veggie water to thin it, if needed. Drink at room temperature for lunch and dinner during the pre-cleanse. Make a fresh batch every day.

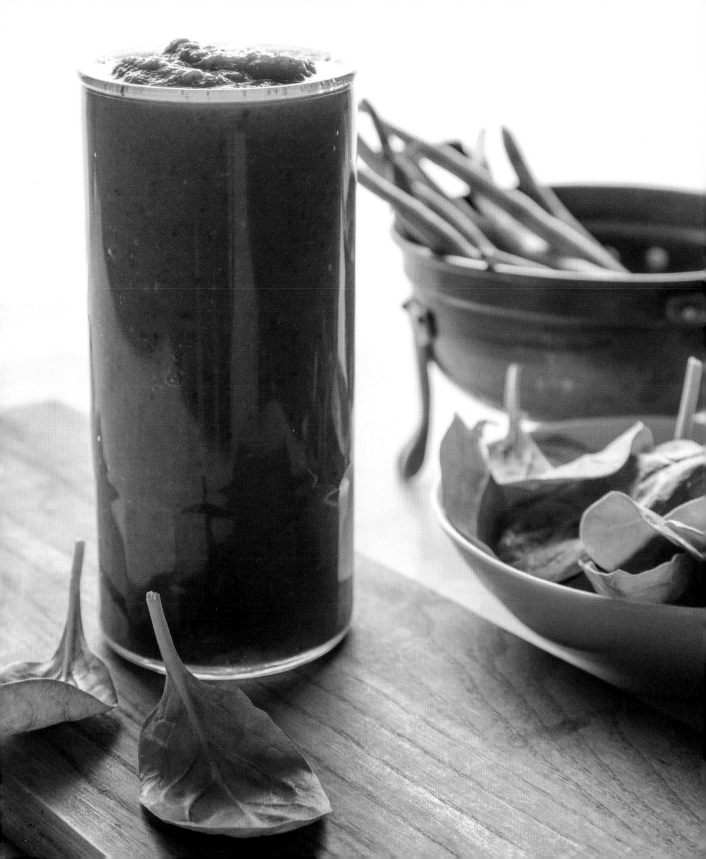

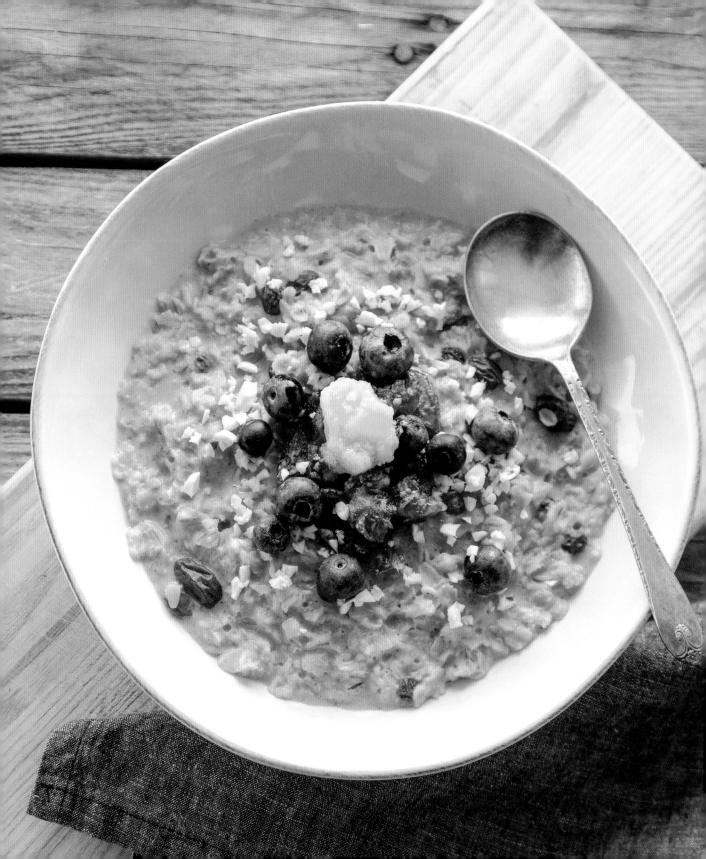

NOT YOUR MOTHER'S OATMEAL

This hearty breakfast is an ideal energy-promoting breakfast and great for Vata and Pitta types as it grounds the central nervous system. Packed with protein and iron, it is sure to keep you going until lunch. Add 1 teaspoon of ghee, and you have added a prebiotic one-two punch for your gut health. This makes two portions, so it is nice to share with a friend or save for another day.

YIELD: 2 servings

10 almonds, soaked overnight

10–15 raisins, soaked overnight in ½ cup (120 ml) water

2 cups (480 ml) almond milk, plus more as needed

1 cup (100 g) rolled oats

¼ tsp ground cardamom

¼ tsp cinnamon powder

¼ tsp ginger powder

¼ tsp vanilla extract (optional)

Pinch of sea salt

½ banana, peeled and sliced (optional)

Handful of blueberries (optional)

2 Medjool dates, chopped (optional)

Ghee or maple syrup, for serving, according to your dosha

Peel the skins off the soaked almonds and chop them. Drain the raisins and retain the raisin water.

In a medium saucepan, bring the almond milk and the raisin water to a boil over medium heat. Pour in the oats, and then add the raisins, almonds, cardamom, cinnamon, ginger, vanilla and salt. Reduce the heat and simmer, stirring occasionally, for about 8 minutes, or until the mixture is smooth and creamy. Stir in the banana, blueberries, dates or fruit of your choice. Serve it in a bowl with extra almond milk, and 1 teaspoon or so of ghee or maple syrup.

Dosha Adaptations

RECIPE WRITTEN FOR VATA.

PITTA: Omit the ginger powder and replace the almond milk with coconut milk.

KAPHA: Use tapioca instead of oatmeal. Replace the almond milk with just 1 cup (240 ml) of soy milk. Cook a little longer to make it dryer and sweeten it with a drizzle of raw honey instead of maple syrup. Omit the ghee.

VEGGIE BREAKFAST TACOS AND SALSA

The high fiber of the beans in this recipe cleanses the small intestine of toxicity as it leads to bulkier stools and more elimination. That's great for Vatas, who tend toward constipation. The high fiber also reduces cholesterol, which Kaphas can have problems with. Meanwhile the adzuki beans are slightly diuretic, flushing and cleansing the urinary tract and kidneys of toxic heat; that's good news for you Pittas that can suffer from overheating. Choose the salsa you prefer.

YIELD: 4 servings

1 (15-oz [430-g]) can adzuki beans, drained and rinsed

8 whole-grain tortillas

Avocado salsa or mango salsa, as desired (see right)

1 cup (60 g) shredded red cabbage

2 tsp (2 g) chopped chives

Preheat the oven to 350°F (180°C).

In a small saucepan, warm the beans over low heat for a minute or two.

Warm the tortillas on a baking sheet in the oven for a minute or two. Place the warm tortillas on plates. Divide the beans among the tortillas. Top them with the avocado or mango salsa and cabbage. Sprinkle the chives and serve.

AVOCADO SALSA

3 ripe Hass avocados, peeled and pitted

½ cup (120 ml) cream

1 cup (240 ml) vegetable broth

1 tsp salt

2 tbsp (30 ml) fresh lime juice

Place the avocados, cream, broth, salt and lime juice in a blender or food processor and process to your desired consistency.

MANGO SALSA

1 large mango, chopped

½ small onion, finely chopped

2 tbsp (30 ml) fresh lime juice, plus more, divided

2 tsp (6 g) dosha-specific spice mix (page 32)

Pinch of asafetida (hing)

¼ tsp salt

¼ tsp pepper

Handful of fresh cilantro, chopped

Lime wedges, for serving

In a medium bowl, toss the mango, onion, lime juice, dosha spice mix, asafetida, salt and pepper. Fold in the cilantro and add a squeeze of lime juice. Garnish with the lime wedges.

Dosha Adaptations

RECIPE WRITTEN FOR VATA.

PITTA: Remove the chives from the tacos, which are too heating, and add chopped cilantro instead.

KAPHA: Avocados are too heavy for Kaphas. Try using steamed cauliflower and non-dairy cream instead.

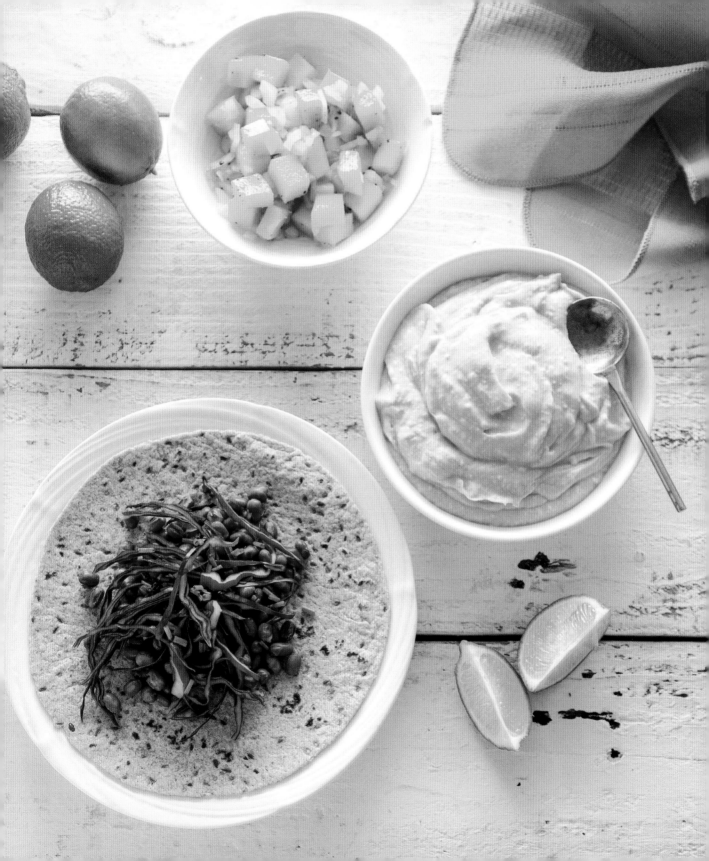

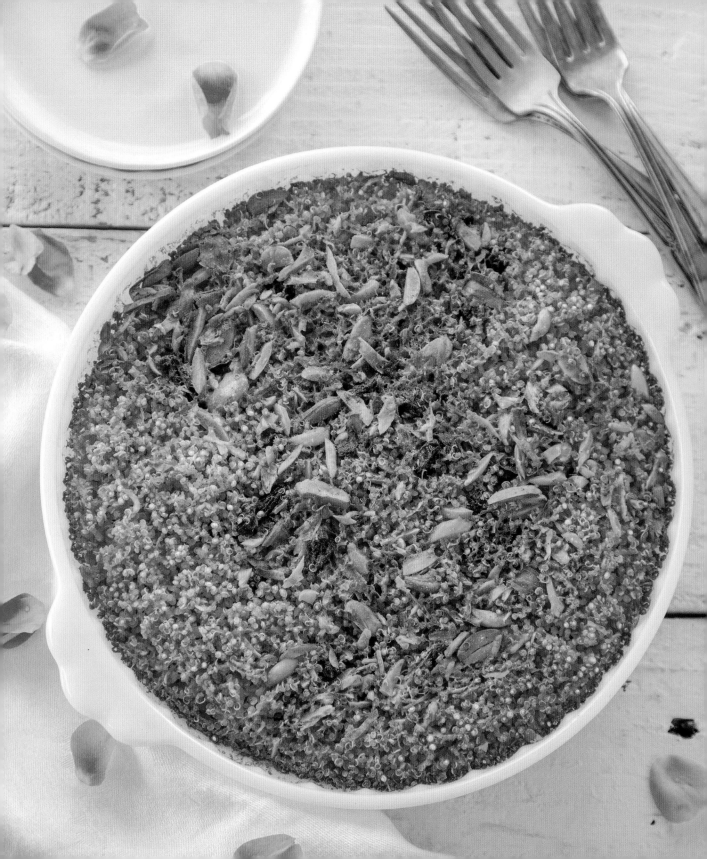

QUINOA BAKE WITH WARM SPICED MILK

Quinoa is a delicious breakfast pseudocereal (more closely related to spinach and beets than to cereals or grains) that's super-high in protein, which benefits all doshas. Combined here with warming, pungent spices, this breakfast bake is satisfying enough to get you through the morning without weighing you down.

YIELD: 4 servings

2 tbsp (30 ml) melted coconut oil, divided

1 cup (180 g) uncooked quinoa, rinsed

2 cups (480 ml) water, plus more as needed

2 cups (480 ml) almond milk

½ tsp ground ginger

1 tsp ground cinnamon

½ tsp ground cardamom

½ cup (70 g) dried raisins (optional)

½ cup (50 g) raw almonds, slivered

Pinch of Himalayan salt

Maple syrup, as desired

Preheat the oven to 350°F (180°C). Coat a baking dish with 1 tablespoon (15 ml) of the coconut oil.

In a medium saucepan, heat the remaining 1 tablespoon (15 ml) of coconut oil over medium-high heat. Add the quinoa and cook, stirring, for about 1 minute, or until the quinoa dries, sizzles and pops. Add the water, reduce the heat and simmer, stirring occasionally, for 15 minutes, or until the quinoa is soft and the mixture thickens. Add more water if needed.

When the quinoa is nearly done, add the almond milk, ginger, cinnamon, cardamom, raisins and almonds in another saucepan. Warm the mixture over low heat.

Transfer the quinoa to the baking dish. Add the salt and pour the almond milk mixture over the top. Sweeten it with maple syrup.

Bake for 50 to 55 minutes, or until cooked through. Remove the dish from the oven and set it aside to cool. Don't worry, the mixture may still be a little watery. Let it stand for about 30 minutes and serve warm.

Dosha Adaptations

RECIPE WRITTEN FOR VATA.

PITTA: Substitute coconut milk for the almond milk and remove the ginger.

KAPHA: Use soy milk instead of almond milk and use raw honey as your sweetener. Try using cranberries instead of raisins.

STEWED PEACHES WITH DATES, CARDAMOM AND ALMOND CREAM

This comforting breakfast is good enough for dessert. It's great for balancing Vata as cooked fruit is really easy to digest and helps keep the body clean. This breakfast has a cooling effect due to the predominance of its sweet taste, so it's an excellent start to any summer's day.

YIELD: 2 servings

2 large peaches, peeled, pitted and sliced

4 Medjool dates, pitted and halved

1½ cups (360 ml) water, divided, plus more as needed

1 tbsp (20 g) maple syrup

1 tsp grated fresh ginger

⅛ tsp ground cardamom

⅛ tsp ground cinnamon

1½ cups (210 g) raw almonds

2 tbsp (40 g) rice syrup

Juice of ½ lemon

In a large saucepan, mix together the peaches, dates, 1 cup (240 ml) of the water, maple syrup, ginger, cardamom and cinnamon and bring it to a boil. Reduce the heat and simmer, covered, for 5 minutes.

Transfer half the mixture to a blender or food processor and process it until pureed. Return it to the pan and stir well.

Place the almonds, remaining ½ cup (120 ml) water, rice syrup and lemon juice in a food processor and process until it's smooth and creamy. Add more water if needed. Serve the peach mixture warmed in bowls with the almond cream mixture drizzled on top.

Dosha Adaptations

RECIPE WRITTEN FOR VATA.

PITTA: Remove the ginger and add 1 tablespoon (5 g) unsweetened coconut flakes when cooking.

KAPHA: Substitute raisins for the dates and add a pinch of cloves.

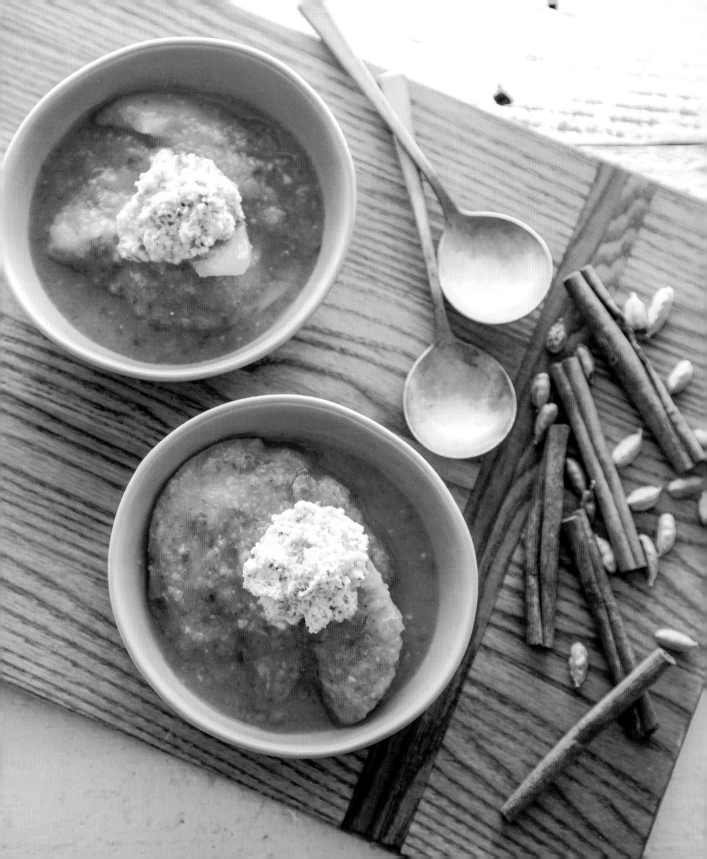

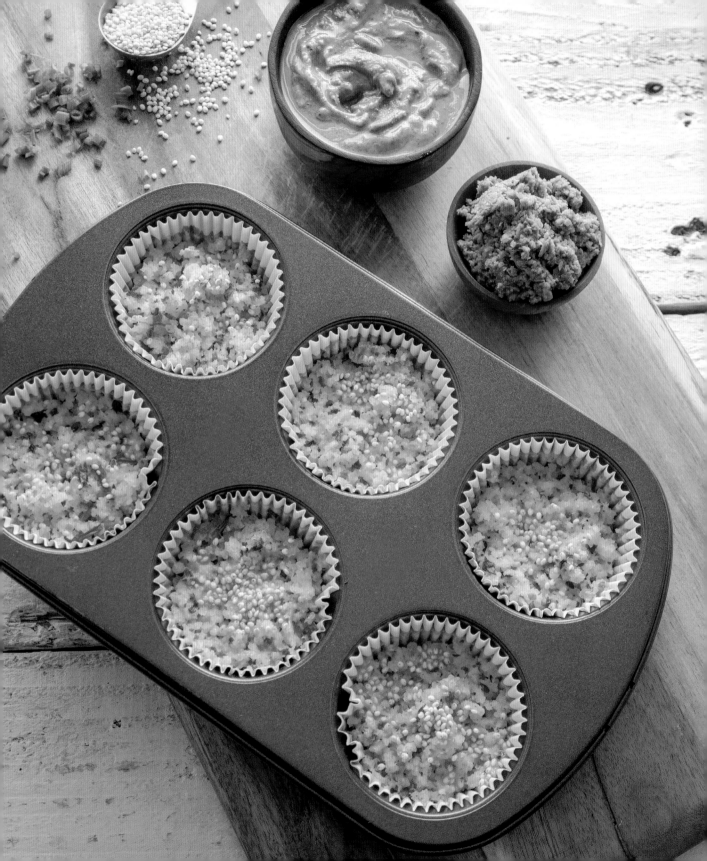

MILLET CAKES WITH NUT BUTTER

Are there some mornings when you fancy something savory? Try millet. It is considered sweet, heating, dry and light. This makes millet a rather special grain because it has the satisfying, nourishing effect of the sweet taste, but it's also light, easy to digest and an antidote to the damp stickiness that can result from eating other, heavier grains (like wheat). Due to its light, heating and drying effect, millet is used in the treatment of high ama (toxins), dull agni (digestive fire), diabetes, excess weight, edema and other excess Kapha (mucous/fluid) conditions. Served with a sweet and spicy nut butter . . . it's delicious! Choose the nut butter according to your dosha (see Dosha Adaptations).

YIELD: 6 servings

1 cup (180 g) cooked millet

1 tbsp (10 g) ground flaxseed

2 cups (480 ml) rice milk

1 tsp minced garlic

¼ cup (12 g) chopped chives

1 tbsp (15 ml) extra-virgin olive oil

Uncooked millet, as desired (optional)

Almond and cashew nut butter or the roasted saffron pumpkin seed butter, as desired (see right).

Preheat the oven to 400°F (200°C). Prepare a 6-cup muffin tin with oil or paper liners.

In a large bowl, stir together the cooked millet, flaxseed, rice milk, garlic, chives and olive oil. Stir to combine them. Set it aside for 5 minutes.

Spoon the millet batter into the prepared tin, filling them two-thirds full. Sprinkle each cup with a little uncooked millet, if desired, and bake for 20 to 25 minutes, or until the muffins are firm and brown on top.

Serve the millet cakes warm with either the almond and cashew nut butter or the roasted saffron pumpkin seed butter. Hint: Make a double batch of nut butter to freeze in order to use it with the Carrot Muffins with Nut Butter (page 154) in the post-cleanse phase.

ALMOND AND CASHEW NUT BUTTER

1 cup (260 g) cashew butter

1 cup (260 g) almond butter

1 tbsp (20 g) maple syrup

1 tsp ground cardamom

½ tsp ground cinnamon

½ tsp vanilla extract

Combine the cashew butter, almond butter, maple syrup, cardamom, cinnamon and vanilla in a food processor. Process until they're thoroughly blended.

ROASTED SAFFRON PUMPKIN SEED BUTTER

2 cups (280 g) raw pumpkin seeds

¼ cup (60 ml) extra-virgin olive oil

1 tbsp (20 g) sweetener (Kaphas: honey; Pittas: maple syrup; Vatas: rice syrup)

Pinch of saffron threads

¼ tsp Himalayan salt

Preheat the oven to 350°F (180°C).

Spread the pumpkin seeds evenly on a baking sheet. Bake, stirring occasionally, for 20 minutes, or until the seeds are evenly roasted. Remove them from the oven and let them cool.

Place the roasted pumpkin seeds, olive oil, sweetener, saffron and salt in a food processor and pulse until the mixture is smooth and thoroughly blended.

Dosha Adaptations

RECIPE WRITTEN FOR VATA.

PITTA: Substitute the cashew butter with another cup (260 g) of almond butter.

KAPHA: The millet cake is perfect when you substitute soy milk for the rice milk.

BREAKFAST RICE

There are a few foods that Ayurveda has established as good for everyone, year-round, and rice is number one on the list. White rice inevitably has less fiber than brown, but it still has nutritional value and provides protein and energy. And since the outer shell of white rice has been removed, it is much easier for Vatas to digest. For this reason, white rice is recommended when digestive ability is low.

YIELD: 2 servings

1 cup (185 g) uncooked white basmati rice

2¼ cups (540 ml) water

⅛ tsp salt

¼ tsp ground coriander

⅛ tsp ground cardamom

1 tsp ghee

In a medium pot, add the rice, water, salt, coriander, cardamom and ghee and bring them to a boil. Reduce the heat to low and simmer for 20 minutes, or until the rice is soft. Serve warm and enjoy.

Dosha Adaptations

RECIPE WRITTEN FOR VATA.
PITTA: No substitutions needed.
KAPHA: No substitutions needed.

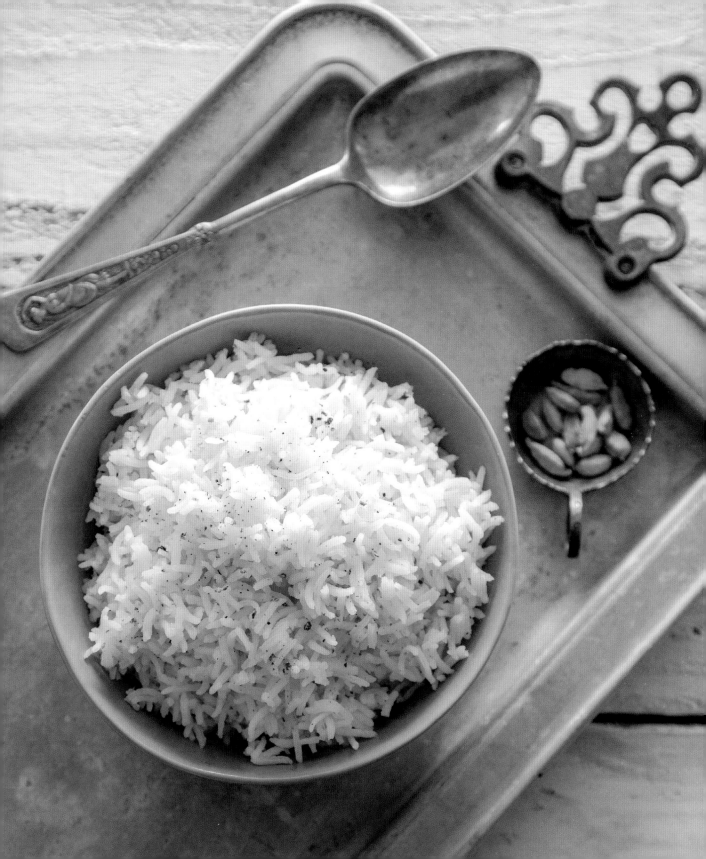

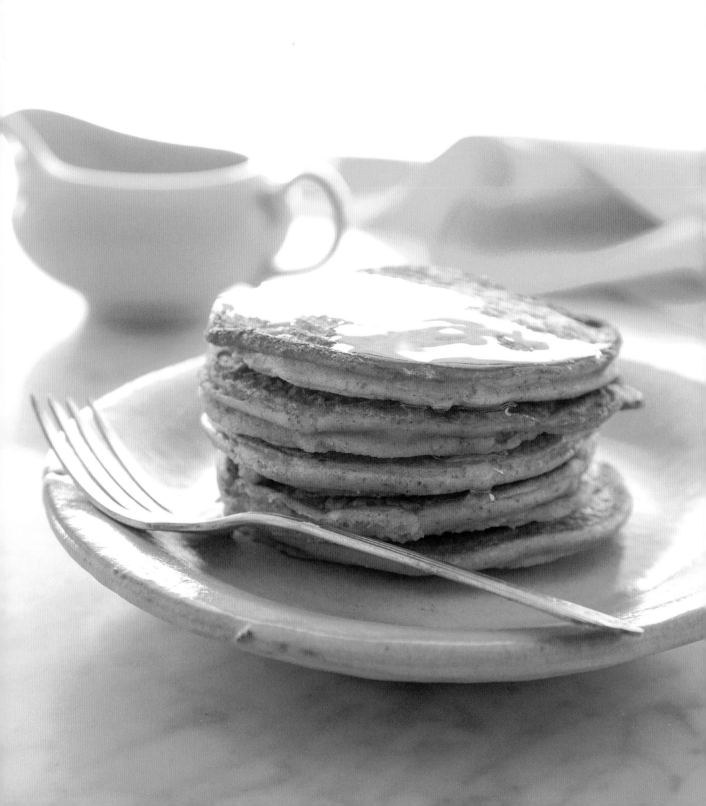

YUMMY BREAKFAST PANCAKES

We made these pancakes with barley flour as it is relatively easier to digest and does not produce excess mucus in the body. Its high insoluble fiber content effectively regulates blood sugar levels. Barley increases the release of bile from the liver and gall bladder, aiding fat metabolism. And as an added bonus, the high-fiber content holds your appetite longer, so you won't find yourself snacking on high-calorie foods. You can purchase egg substitutes at the grocery store.

YIELD: 4 servings

1 cup (140 g) barley flour

¼ tsp salt

1 tsp baking powder

½ ripe avocado, pitted and peeled

1 egg substitute

1½ cups (360 ml) water

½ tsp cinnamon

⅛ tsp ground nutmeg

¼ tsp ghee, plus more as desired

In a small bowl, mix together the barley flour, salt and baking powder. Set it aside.

In a blender, add the avocado, egg substitute, water, cinnamon and nutmeg and process until it's smooth. Add this mixture to the barley mixture and combine them to form a batter.

Heat a skillet over medium heat and add the ghee. When hot, pour enough batter into the skillet to form a small circle. When the batter begins to bubble and brown, about 1 to 2 minutes, flip it and cook the other side. Place the pancake on a warming plate. Repeat until all the batter is gone. Serve them hot with more ghee.

Dosha Adaptations

RECIPE WRITTEN FOR VATA.
PITTA: No substitutions needed.
KAPHA: No substitutions needed.

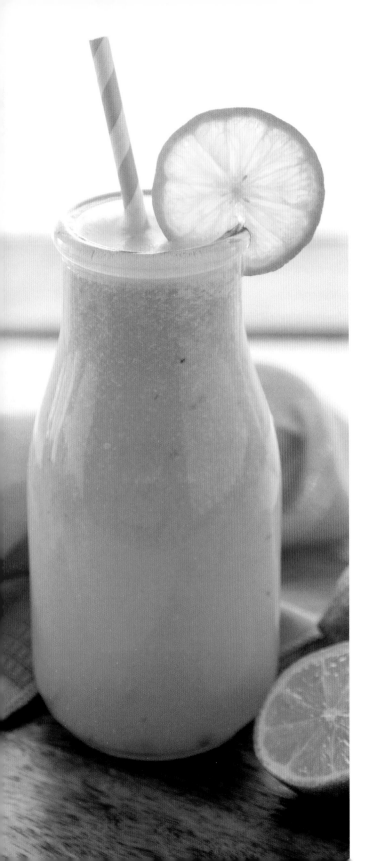

COCONUT CUCUMBER SMOOTHIE

This cooling and refreshing breakfast drink is great for those days when your digestive fire is a little low, which tends to happen in the summer. However, you will still need something nutritious that will sustain you throughout your morning. This smoothie will be ideal, as it cools Pitta and pacifies Vata. Try adding some almond butter if you feel in need of more protein.

YIELD: 2 servings

2 cups (480 ml) coconut water
2 cucumbers, peeled
2 tbsp (30 ml) lime juice
1 tbsp (15 g) almond butter (optional)

In a blender, add the coconut water, cucumbers, lime juice and almond butter (if using) and process until it's smooth and creamy. Drink immediately.

Dosha Adaptations
RECIPE WRITTEN FOR VATA.
PITTA: No substitutions needed.
KAPHA: Omit the almond butter.

STIMULATING JUICE COCKTAIL

Freshly prepared vegetable juice makes for an energizing start to the day. This cocktail is particularly excellent for Kaphas, who can feel sluggish first thing in the morning.

YIELD: 2 servings

2 peaches, pitted and chopped
2 carrots, sliced
1 small beet, sliced
½ cup (120 ml) water
2 tbsp (30 ml) coconut milk
2 parsley sprigs

In a blender, add the peaches, carrots, beet, water, coconut milk and parsley and process until it's smooth and creamy.

Dosha Adaptations

RECIPE WRITTEN FOR VATA.
PITTA: Substitute mango for the peaches and a sprig of mint instead of parsley.
KAPHA: Substitute soy milk for the coconut milk.

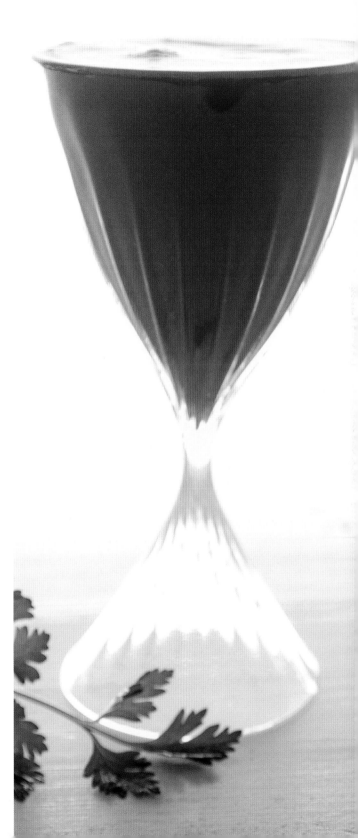

UPMA

Upma is a hot, savory cereal that is quite delicious. It is made by cooking spices in ghee to release their healing qualities. Dry-roasting the grains removes the allergens from wheat and makes it easily digestible. Balancing for all three doshas, it's a great breakfast especially in fall or spring when allergies are likely to run high.

YIELD: 4 servings

1 cup (180 g) cream of wheat cereal (farina)

1 tbsp (15 g) ghee

1 tsp black mustard seed

½ tsp ground turmeric

2 green chiles, seeded and chopped

1 onion, chopped

¼ cup (10 g) cilantro leaves, chopped, plus extra for garnishing

½ tsp salt

3 cups (720 ml) water

1 tsp lemon juice

⅓ cup (20 g) unsweetened coconut flakes

In a medium saucepan, dry-roast the cream of wheat for 5 minutes, or until it begins to brown. Stir frequently so it doesn't burn. Remove it from the heat and set it aside.

In a large saucepan, melt the ghee, add the mustard seed and cook until the seeds pop. Stir in the turmeric, chiles, onion and cilantro and cook for 8 to 10 minutes, or until the onion is slightly browned. Add the salt and water and bring it to a boil. Add the cream of wheat while stirring continuously to avoid lumps. Cook for 2 minutes. Reduce the heat and simmer for another 5 minutes, or until cooked through. Turn off the heat. Stir in the lemon juice and garnish with coconut flakes and some more cilantro.

Dosha Adaptations

RECIPE WRITTEN FOR VATA.
PITTA: No substitutions needed.
KAPHA: Omit the coconut flakes, add a chopped clove of garlic with the onion and add more chiles.

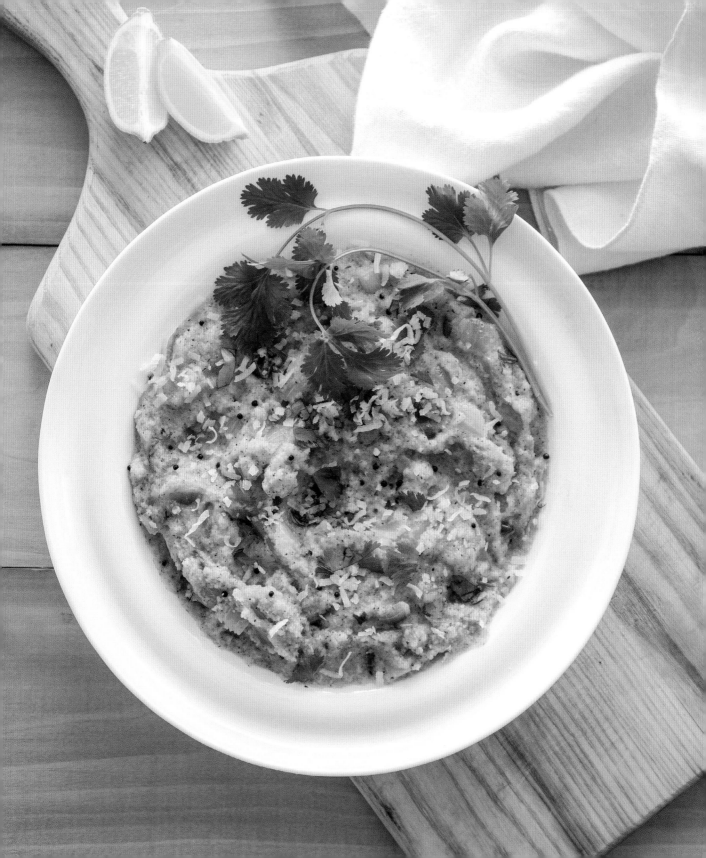

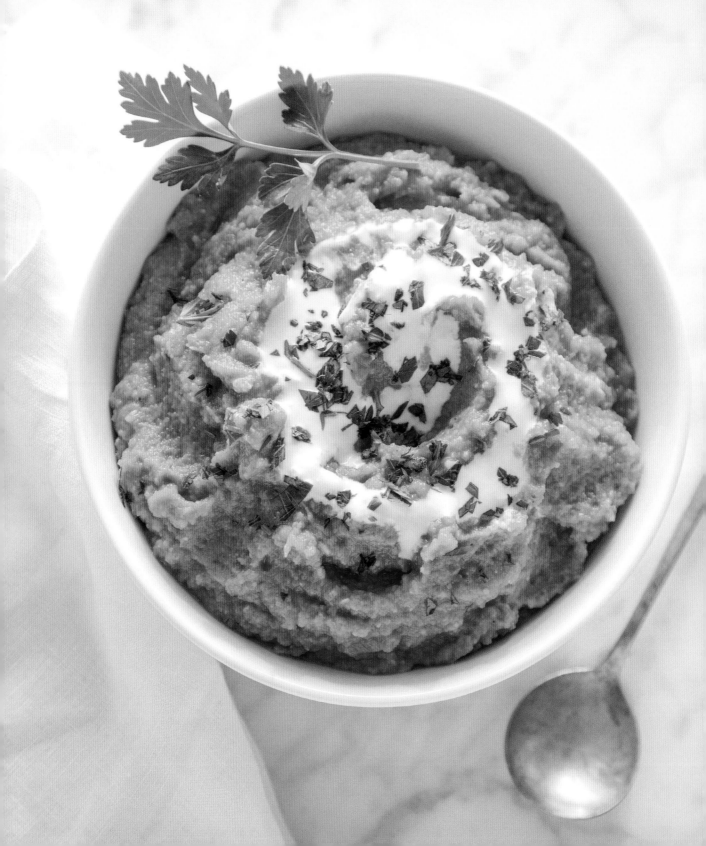

DETOX BREAKFAST STEW

This stew is packed with potassium, for creating an alkaline environment, and helps flush out the toxins from our cells, as well as adding fiber, for stimulating bile secretion and promoting bowel movement and elimination of toxins. This stew will make you feel amazing.

YIELD: 2 servings

1 sweet potato, peeled and cubed

3 carrots, peeled and roughly chopped

1 parsnip, peeled and roughly chopped

1 onion, peeled and cut in quarters

3 cloves garlic, crushed

¼ tsp sea salt

Pinch of chili powder

1 tsp turmeric powder

1 tsp cumin powder

1 tbsp (14 g) coconut oil

2 cups (480 ml) low-sodium vegetable broth, warmed

½" (12-mm) piece ginger, peeled and grated

½ cup (100 g) cooked red lentils

Fresh parsley, for garnishing

1 tsp coconut milk, for garnishing

Preheat the oven to 325°F (165°C). Line a baking sheet with parchment paper.

In a large bowl, add the sweet potato, carrots, parsnip, onion, garlic, salt, chili powder, turmeric, cumin and coconut oil and toss to combine them. Spread the mixture on the baking sheet and roast for 20 minutes, or until they're browned.

Transfer the roasted veggie mix to a blender. Add the warm vegetable broth, ginger and lentils and process until the mixture resembles a smooth cream. Serve warm, garnished with parsley and a drizzle of coconut milk.

Dosha Adaptations

RECIPE WRITTEN FOR VATA.

PITTA: Remove the chili powder.

KAPHA: Use sunflower oil instead of coconut oil.

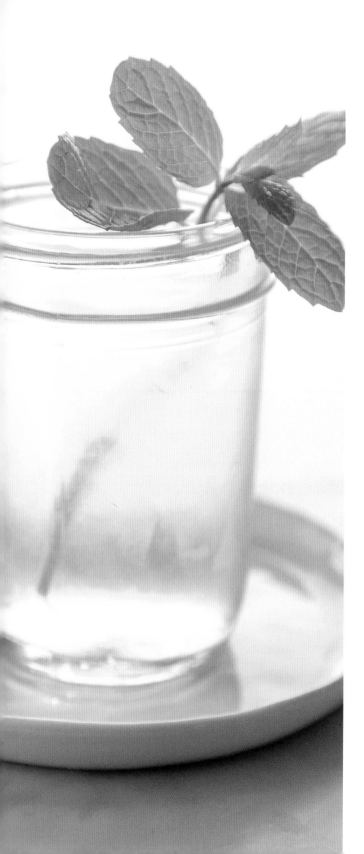

MINT TEA

This tea is soothing to the digestive system and especially cooling for Pittas or in Pitta season (summer).

YIELD: 2 servings

2 cups (480 ml) filtered water
20 fresh mint leaves, chopped

In a saucepan, bring the water to a boil over medium heat. Add the mint leaves, steep for 5 minutes and then drain the leaves. Pour the tea through a tea strainer. Serve either hot or at room temperature.

Dosha Adaptations

RECIPE WRITTEN FOR VATA.
PITTA: This recipe is recommended to be served cool.
KAPHA: This recipe is recommended to be served hot.

GINGER TEA

This is a great tea for when you're feeling a little nauseated or your tummy is hurting. It's really good for Kaphas and Vatas in Kapha season (late winter and spring).

YIELD: 2 servings

2 cups (480 ml) filtered water
1" (2.5-cm) piece ginger, peeled and grated
1 tsp freshly squeezed lemon juice (optional)
Raw honey, as desired (optional)

In a saucepan, bring the water to a boil over medium heat. Add the ginger and simmer for 3 to 5 minutes over low heat. Remove the pan from the heat. Strain and add the lemon juice and raw honey if needed. Serve hot.

Dosha Adaptations

RECIPE WRITTEN FOR VATA.
PITTA: This recipe is recommended to be served cool with lime juice instead of lemon.
KAPHA: This recipe is recommended to be served hot.

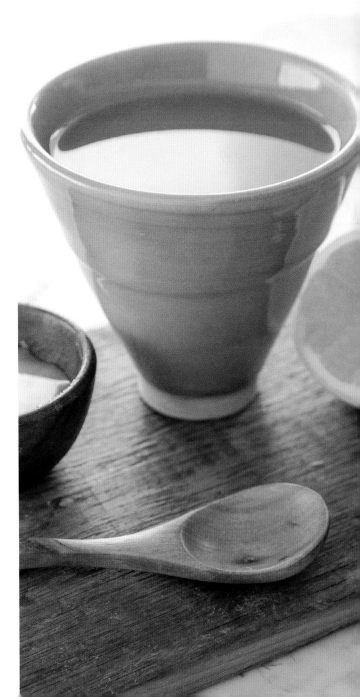

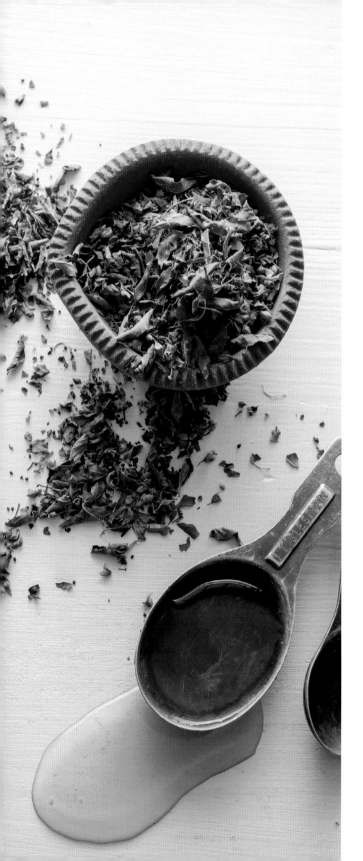

TULSI TEA

Sipping on this tea improves digestion and removes congestion. So, if you suffer from sinus congestion, lung congestion or even blood congestion (cholesterol)—this is the tea for you. It's especially good during Kapha season (late winter and spring).

YIELD: 2 servings

2 cups (480 ml) filtered water
1" (2.5-cm) piece ginger, peeled and grated
1 cup (12 g) tulsi leaves (holy basil)
Raw honey or raw cane sugar, as desired (optional)

In a saucepan, bring the water to a boil over medium heat. Add the ginger, reduce the heat to low and simmer for 2 minutes. Add the tulsi and simmer for 3 minutes. Remove it from the heat and let it steep for 5 minutes. Strain and serve with honey or raw cane sugar, if needed. Serve it hot.

Dosha Adaptations

RECIPE WRITTEN FOR VATA.
PITTA: Substitute a sprig of fresh mint for the ginger.
KAPHA: This recipe is recommended to be served hot.

DANDELION TEA

This is a terrific tea for liver cleansing and a must-have tea while on your cleanse. It's good for all doshas in all seasons.

YIELD: 2 servings

2 cups (480 ml) filtered water

2 cardamom pods

1 cup (20 g) dandelion leaves

Freshly squeezed lemon juice, as desired (optional)

Raw honey, as desired (optional)

In a saucepan, bring the water to a boil over medium heat. Add the cardamom pods, return it to a boil and simmer for 5 minutes. Add the dandelion leaves and steep it for 5 minutes, or to taste. Strain and serve it warm with a squeeze of lemon juice and/or honey, if needed.

Dosha Adaptations

RECIPE WRITTEN FOR VATA.

PITTA: This recipe is recommended to be served at room temperature.

KAPHA: This recipe is recommended to be served hot.

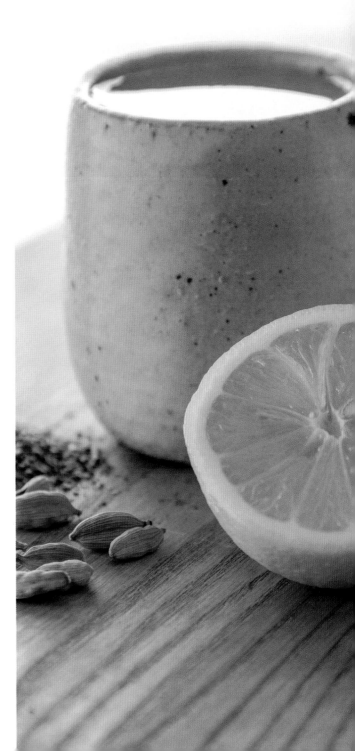

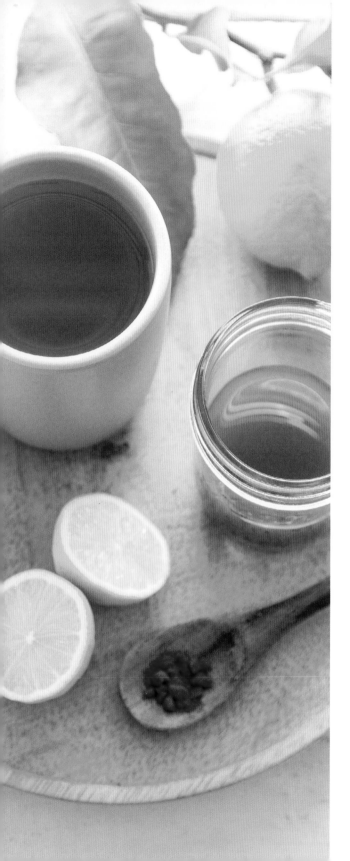

AGNI-BOOSTING TEA

Drink this tea before meals for its agni-promoting benefits as well as for its ability to jump-start your metabolism in a natural and gentle way. If you have any symptoms of heartburn, diarrhea or acidity—this tea is too heating for you.

YIELD: 2 servings

2 tbsp (30 ml) apple cider vinegar

Pinch of cayenne pepper

2 tbsp (30 ml) lemon juice

Honey, as desired (optional)

2 cups (480 ml) filtered water, boiled and slightly cooled

In a mug, combine the apple cider vinegar, cayenne pepper, lemon juice and honey (if using). Pour in the water. Stir and slowly sip. Serve hot.

Dosha Adaptations

RECIPE WRITTEN FOR VATA.

PITTA: Do not drink if there are any symptoms of heartburn or acidity.

KAPHA: This drink is recommended to be served hot.

DIGESTIVE TEA

This fennel tea is designed to reduce any heat in the body while simultaneously working on your agni with the cinnamon and ginger. Calming for even that finicky Vata digestion, this tea utilizes the slipperiness of licorice to combat any dryness—especially in Vata season (fall and early winter).

YIELD: 2 servings

1" (2.5-cm) piece ginger, peeled and chopped

1 tbsp (9 g) fennel seeds

1 cinnamon stick

2 tsp (6 g) licorice root or the contents of 2 licorice tea bags

1 tbsp (3 g) dried mint

2 cups (480 ml) filtered water

Lime juice, as desired

Liquid stevia or honey, as desired (optional)

Place the ginger, fennel, cinnamon, licorice and mint in a teapot.

In a saucepan, boil the water and pour it into the teapot. Let it steep for 10 minutes. Pour it into a mug and add a squeeze of lime. Sweeten with liquid stevia or drizzle with a little honey, if needed.

Dosha Adaptations
RECIPE WRITTEN FOR VATA.
PITTA: No substitutions needed.
KAPHA: No substitutions needed.

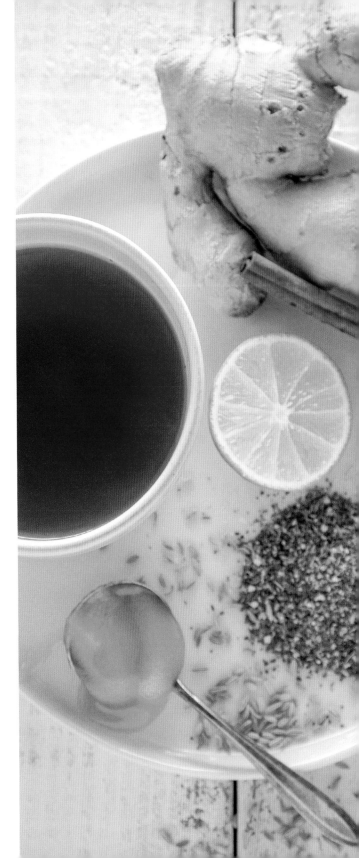

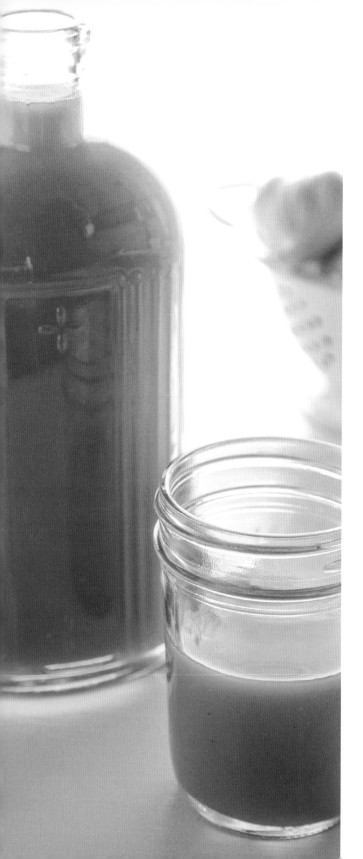

BREAKTIME BENEFICIAL BROTH

Feeling a little sluggish? Take a break and sip on this broth for its energizing and calming qualities. Good for all doshas.

YIELD: 1 serving

1 cup (240 ml) vegetable broth or stock
1 tsp dosha-specific spice mix (page 32)

In a saucepan, bring the vegetable broth to a boil. Add the dosha spice mix, lower the heat and simmer gently for 3 minutes. Pour it into a cup or flask and sip it throughout the day.

Dosha Adaptations
RECIPE WRITTEN FOR VATA.
PITTA: Add the Pitta spice mix.
KAPHA: Add the Kapha spice mix.

SAFFRON LEMONADE

A cooling and incredibly sattvic (fresh, juicy and light) drink that leaves you feeling refreshed and rejuvenated. Best to drink in Pitta season (summer).

YIELD: 1 serving

Water, to fill a saucepan halfway

Pinch of saffron threads

Juice of 1 lemon

1 cup (240 ml) sparkling mineral water

Sprig of mint, for garnishing

Liquid stevia or other liquid sweetener, as desired (optional)

Bring a saucepan half full of water to a boil. Place the saffron in a small bowl and heat the bowl over the boiling water for 2 to 3 minutes. Remove the bowl from the heat and with the back of a spoon, press the saffron to break up the threads. Remove the water from the heat and add 2 tablespoons (30 ml) of warm water to the saffron. Set it aside for 20 minutes.

Add the lemon juice and mineral water to the bowl. Garnish with the mint and add a sweetener if needed. Pour it into a glass and drink immediately.

Dosha Adaptations

RECIPE WRITTEN FOR VATA.
PITTA: No substitutions needed.
KAPHA: No substitutions needed.

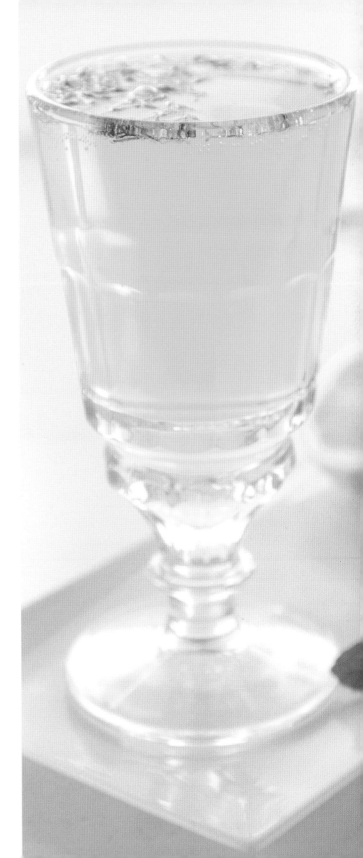

CLEANSING BUDDHA BOWL

Here's a flavorful, protein-packed lunch that is very satisfying. Freekeh is a supergrain made from green durum wheat. Turmeric is good at moving stagnation in the blood and reducing pathogenic bacteria. Serve with the dressing of your choice (see right).

YIELD: 2 servings

2 cups (182 g) broccoli florets

2 cups (268 g) asparagus, trimmed and cut into 2″ (5-cm) pieces

8 baby red potatoes, washed and sliced

1 cup (122 g) sliced carrots

3 oz (85 g) seasoned and cooked tempeh, thinly sliced

2 tbsp (30 ml) extra-virgin olive oil or avocado oil

Salt and pepper, as desired

1 cup (200 g) cooked freekeh

2 cups (60 g) baby spinach

¼ cup (15 g) shredded purple cabbage

1 avocado, peeled, pitted and chopped

Turmeric dressing or green tahini dressing, as desired (see right)

Preheat the oven to 425°F (220°C). Line a baking sheet with parchment paper.

Arrange the broccoli, asparagus, potatoes, carrots and tempeh on the baking sheet. Drizzle evenly with the oil and season well with salt and pepper. Place the sheet in the oven and roast for 18 to 20 minutes, or until the vegetables are tender and just beginning to brown.

To serve, place the freekeh and spinach evenly into two shallow bowls. Divide the veggies and tempeh between the bowls. Add the purple cabbage and avocado. Spoon on the dressing and serve immediately.

TURMERIC DRESSING

2 cups (480 g) coconut cream

2 tbsp (30 g) tahini

Juice of 1 lemon

1 tsp ground turmeric

¼ tsp sea salt

¼ tsp black pepper

In a small bowl, whisk together the cream, tahini, lemon juice, turmeric, salt and pepper. Store it in an airtight container in the refrigerator for up to 1 week.

GREEN TAHINI DRESSING

Juice of 1½ lemons

1 clove garlic, minced

2 tbsp (30 g) tahini

¼ cup (10 g) chopped parsley

2 tbsp (30 ml) extra-virgin olive oil

1–3 tbsp (15–45 ml) water

Salt and pepper, as desired

In a food processor or blender, process the lemon juice, garlic, tahini, parsley and olive oil. Add up to 3 tablespoons (45 ml) of water to achieve a thinner consistency. Season with salt and pepper and store it in an airtight container in the refrigerator for up to a week.

Dosha Adaptations

RECIPE WRITTEN FOR VATA.

PITTA: No substitutions needed.

KAPHA: Add 1 teaspoon of red pepper flakes and a pinch of paprika to the Turmeric Dressing. Omit the avocado.

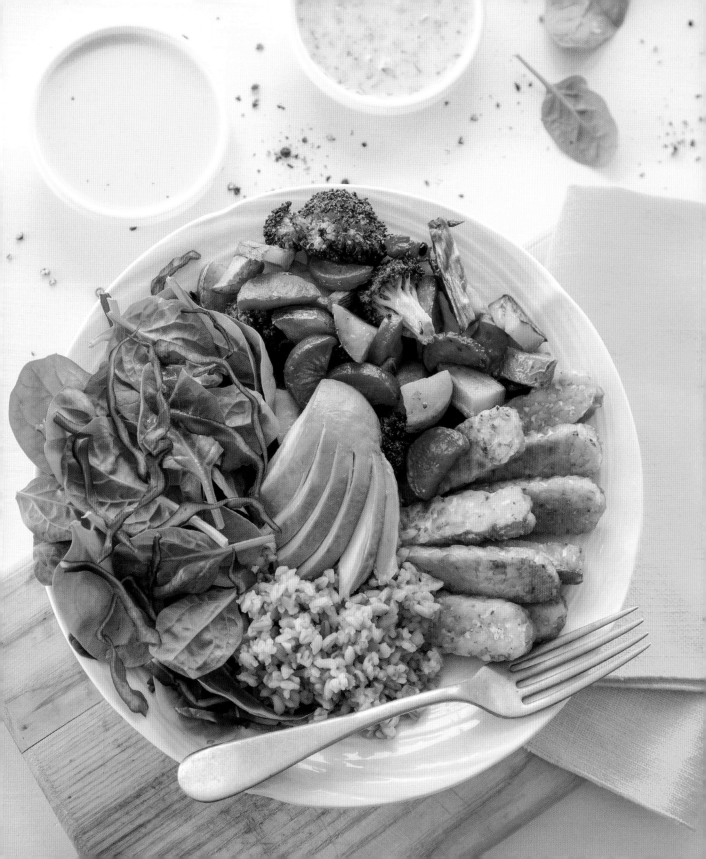

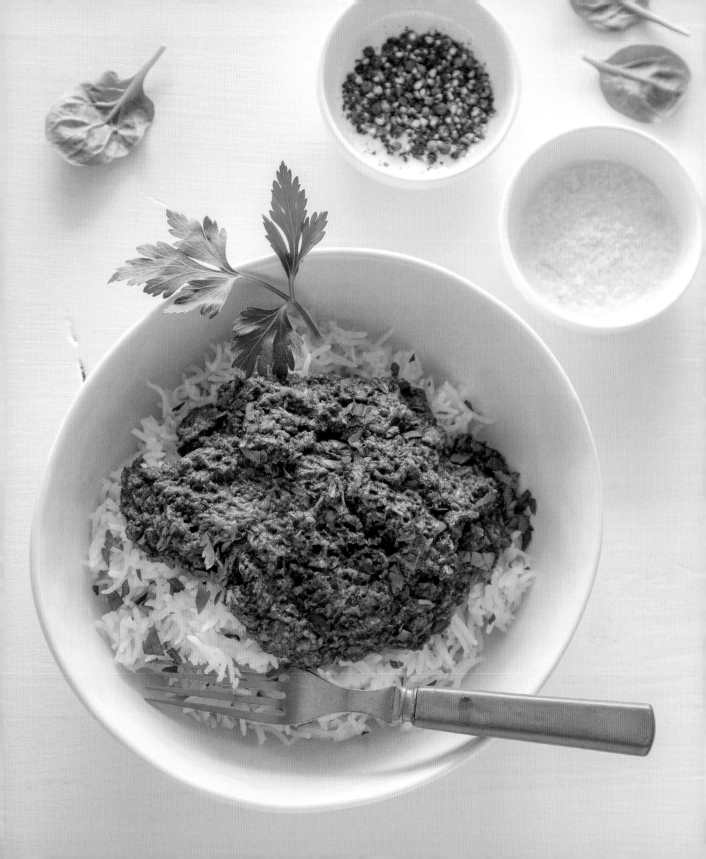

SUMPTUOUS SPINACH CURRY

Peas are a low-fat food and are very important for improving the absorption of proteins, fats and carbohydrates. Peas can help you stay regular and feel satisfied after meals, and they are also high in antioxidants and anti-inflammatory nutrients. This means protection from oxidation damage and certain cancers.

YIELD: 2 servings

1 lb (455 g) chopped frozen spinach, thawed

10 oz (280 g) sweet peas

2 cups (480 ml) vegetable broth or stock

2 tsp (6 g) dosha-specific spice mix (page 32)

2 tsp (6 g) curry powder

1 tsp ground cumin

1 tsp ghee

Salt and pepper, as desired

2 cups (372 g) cooked rice

Fresh parsley, chopped, as desired

In a large skillet, combine the spinach, sweet peas, vegetable broth, dosha spice mix, curry powder, cumin and ghee. Bring it to a boil and simmer for 10 to 15 minutes, or until the vegetables are well cooked.

Allow the mixture to cool and then transfer it to a blender and process until smooth. Season it with salt and pepper.

Transfer the mixture back to the skillet and bring it back to a boil. Turn off the heat and serve over the cooked rice. Garnish it with the parsley.

Dosha Adaptations

RECIPE WRITTEN FOR VATA.

PITTA: Remove the curry powder and add another teaspoon of Pitta spice mix.

KAPHA: No substitutions needed.

EASY VEGETABLE STEW

Winter squashes, including butternut, are eaten in the autumn after they have absorbed the sun's energy over the summer. This stored energy gives squashes a warm ojas (vitality) heartiness that can comfort you through colder weather. Squashes are unusual in that they are not only hearty, but they also drain excess fluids because of their mild diuretic nature. This dual quality makes them ideal for those trying to lose weight but still struggle with comfort-food cravings.

YIELD: 2 servings

1 tbsp (15 g) ghee

1 tsp cumin seeds

½ tsp mustard seeds

4 cloves garlic, grated

1" (2.5-cm) piece ginger, peeled and grated

2 onions, diced

1 green chile, seeded and chopped

2 small zucchinis, diced

1 small butternut squash, peeled and chopped into bite-size chunks

2 tsp (6 g) dosha-specific spice mix (page 32)

1 tsp ground turmeric

1 (14-oz [400-g]) can chickpeas, drained

Salt and pepper, as desired

Preheat a large skillet or wok. Add the ghee, cumin and mustard seeds and cook until the seeds sizzle and pop. Reduce the heat, add the garlic and ginger and cook for 1 minute over medium heat. Add the onions and chile and cook for 3 minutes, or until the onions become translucent.

Add the zucchinis, squash, dosha spice mix and turmeric. Reduce the heat to low and simmer for approximately 15 minutes, covered. Remove the lid, add the chickpeas and simmer for 5 minutes, or until the squash is cooked. Season with the salt and pepper and serve in soup bowls.

Dosha Adaptations

RECIPE WRITTEN FOR VATA.
PITTA: Omit the chile and reduce the garlic to 2 cloves.
KAPHA: Substitute eggplant for the butternut squash.

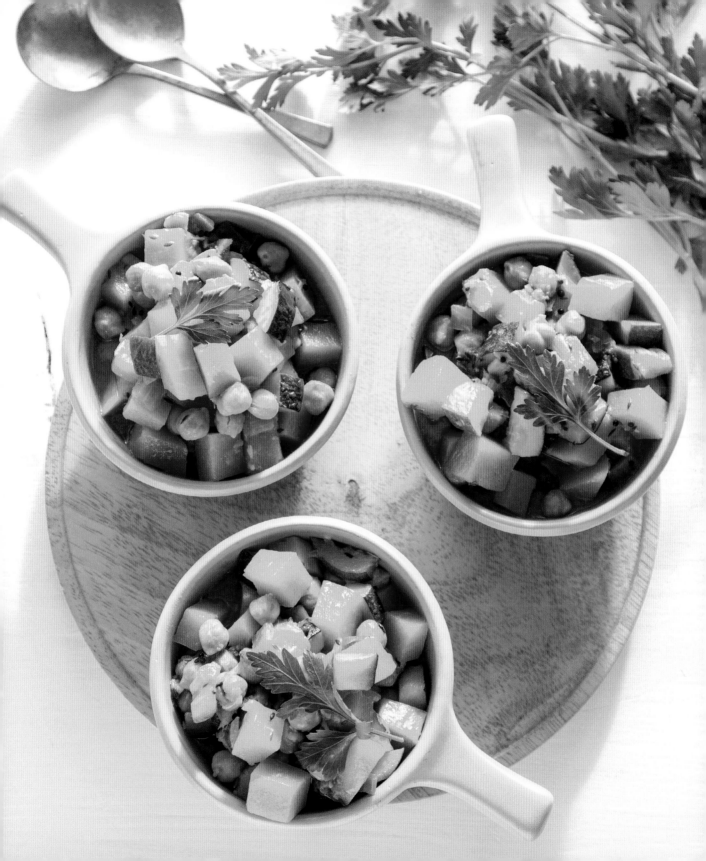

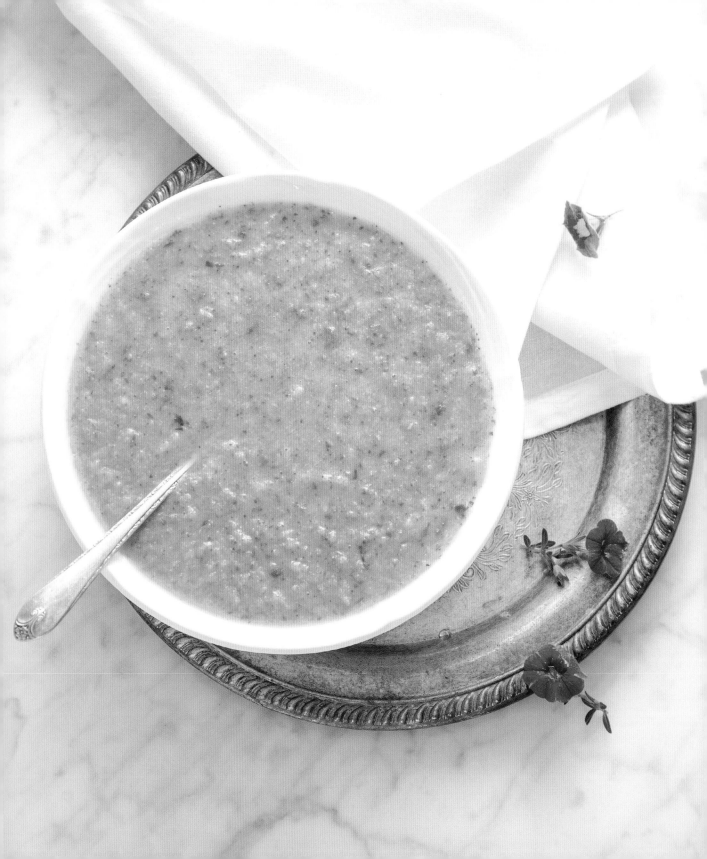

ANTI-INFLAMMATORY BROCCOLI SOUP

Here's a gorgeous, brightly colored detoxifying soup simply loaded with vitamins and minerals.

YIELD: 2 servings

1 tsp ghee

1 onion, finely diced

2 cloves garlic, crushed

1 carrot, peeled and finely chopped

1 parsnip, peeled and finely chopped

2 celery ribs, finely diced

2 cups (182 g) broccoli florets

2 cups (480 ml) filtered water or low-sodium vegetable broth

1 cup (20 g) greens (kale, spinach, beet greens or any other available)

1 tbsp (15 g) chia seeds

½ tsp sea salt

Juice from ½ lemon

In a soup pot, heat the ghee, and then add the onion, garlic, carrot, parsnip, celery and broccoli and cook over low heat for 5 minutes, stirring frequently. Add the water or vegetable broth, bring it to a boil and then cover it and simmer for 5 to 7 minutes, or until the vegetables are tender but not mushy.

Stir in the greens, and then transfer it to a blender. Add the chia seeds, salt and lemon juice and process to obtain a smooth cream. Serve warm.

Dosha Adaptations

RECIPE WRITTEN FOR VATA.

PITTA: No substitutions needed.

KAPHA: No substitutions needed.

ROASTED VEGETABLE BOWL

Grains such as farro help with lubrication, energy, physical strength and endurance. Ayurveda recommends having grains at each meal to provide adequate energy for the body. Vata and Pitta types can consume high quantities of grains, while Kapha types should have smaller amounts to avoid weight gain.

YIELD: 4 servings

1½ cups (300 g) uncooked semi-pearled farro

2 cups (280 g) cubed butternut squash

2 cups (140 g) quartered baby bella mushrooms

2 cups (176 g) quartered or halved Brussels sprouts

6 tbsp (90 g) ghee, divided

Salt and pepper, as desired

Juice of 1½ lemons

1 clove garlic, minced

2 tbsp (30 g) tahini

¼ cup (10 g) fresh parsley leaves

Preheat the oven to 425°F (220°C) and cover two baking sheets with aluminum foil.

Place the farro in a large saucepan and cover it with cold water. Soak the farro for 15 minutes, and then drain it. Return the farro to the pan and cover it again with water. Bring it to a boil and let it simmer for 15 minutes. Drain and spread the farro out on a paper towel–lined plate to cool. Set it aside.

Arrange the squash, mushrooms and Brussels sprouts on the prepared baking sheets and drizzle with 3 tablespoons (45 g) of the ghee. Season with salt and pepper and toss to coat it. Place the sheets in the oven and roast for 15 to 18 minutes, or until the vegetables are golden and tender. Remove them from the oven and let them cool slightly.

In a food processor or blender, combine the lemon juice, garlic, tahini, parsley and remaining 3 tablespoons (45 g) ghee. Process until it's smooth. Add up to 3 tablespoons (45 ml) of water to achieve a thinner consistency, if needed. Season with more salt and pepper.

In a large bowl, toss together the farro and roasted vegetables. Divide them into serving bowls and drizzle with the dressing.

Dosha Adaptations

RECIPE WRITTEN FOR VATA.

PITTA: Use pumpkin seed or sesame seed tahini.

KAPHA: Use pumpkin seed or sunflower seed tahini.

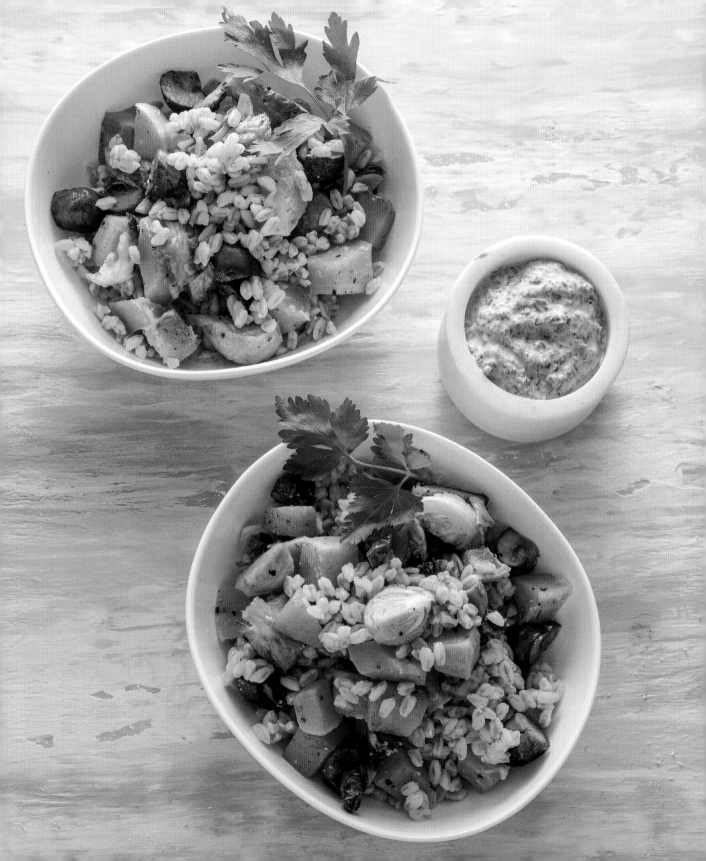

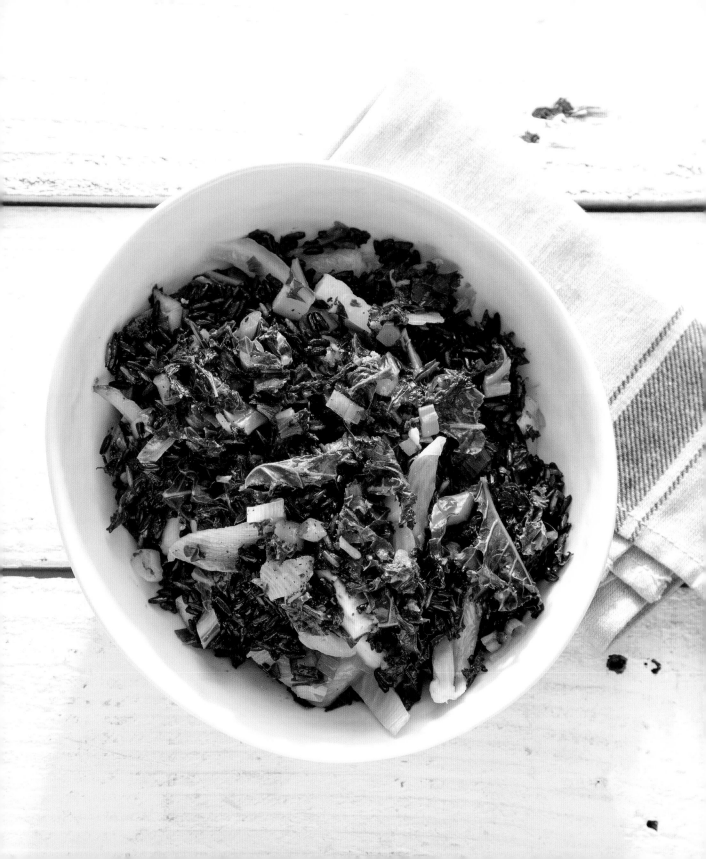

BRAISED KALE AND WILD RICE SALAD WITH FENNEL

Fennel is used as a digestive tonic and a mild laxative. It also helps remove toxins from the body as well as reduce rheumatism and swelling. Certain elements of the essential oils in fennel are stimulants that promote the secretion of digestive and gastric juices, which help reduce inflammation of the stomach and intestines and aid in the proper absorption of nutrients from food.

YIELD: 2 servings

¼ cup (60 ml) lemon or lime juice

2 cloves garlic, minced, divided

¼ cup (60 ml) extra-virgin olive oil

Salt, as desired, divided

2 cups (372 g) cooked wild rice

1 tbsp (15 g) ghee

2 tsp (6 g) grated ginger

½ large fennel bulb, chopped

1 bunch curly or flat-leaf kale

½ cup (24 g) chopped scallions

Pepper, as desired

In a small bowl, combine the lemon or lime juice, 1 clove garlic, olive oil and salt to make the dressing.

In a large bowl, mix together the dressing and the cooked wild rice and set this aside.

In a large skillet, melt the ghee over medium heat. Add the ginger and remaining 1 clove garlic and sauté for 2 to 3 minutes, or until the garlic is translucent. Add the fennel and sauté for 2 to 3 minutes. Add the kale and scallions and sauté for 3 minutes. Add the wild rice to the greens and season with salt and pepper. Serve warm.

Dosha Adaptations

RECIPE WRITTEN FOR VATA.

PITTA: Use lime juice and omit the scallions.

KAPHA: Use sunflower oil instead of olive oil. Add a pinch of red pepper flakes to the dressing.

CHERMOULA AND PASTA

Chermoula is a spice-infused, North African herb sauce that's a staple of Moroccan cuisine. It is traditionally made with cilantro, garlic, coriander, smoked paprika, chili paste, lemon and olive oil. Chermoula has powerful detoxifying properties thanks to the cilantro, which binds to heavy metals and carries them out of the body. Use chermoula as a marinade or spoon it liberally over wild fish, grass-fed steaks, grilled lamb and roasted chicken (after the cleanse)—or enjoy it just as it is in this meal, over pasta.

YIELD: 4 servings

1 tsp cumin seeds

¼ cup (10 g) coarsely chopped flat-leaf parsley

⅓ cup (15 g) coarsely chopped cilantro leaves and tender stems

3 cloves garlic, peeled and chopped

1 tsp smoked paprika

2 tsp (10 ml) fresh lemon juice, divided

6 tbsp (90 ml) extra-virgin olive oil, plus more as needed

½ tsp salt

½ tsp chili paste (or ½–1 fresh chile, seeded and chopped)

1 (16-oz [455-g]) box fusilli pasta (or your favorite dry pasta)

In a skillet, toast the cumin seeds over medium-high heat, stirring, for 1 to 2 minutes, or until they smell fragrant.

In a food processor, add the parsley, cilantro, garlic, smoked paprika, 1 teaspoon of the lemon juice, olive oil, salt, chili paste and toasted cumin. Process until it's smooth.

Add the additional remaining 1 teaspoon of lemon juice and extra olive oil (if needed), until the mixture is a smooth paste.

Cook the pasta until it's al dente according to the package directions. Add the chermoula to the pasta like a pesto. You can keep the chermoula refrigerated for about 3 days.

Dosha Adaptations

RECIPE WRITTEN FOR VATA.
PITTA: Omit the smoked paprika and chili paste.
KAPHA: Substitute canola oil for the olive oil.

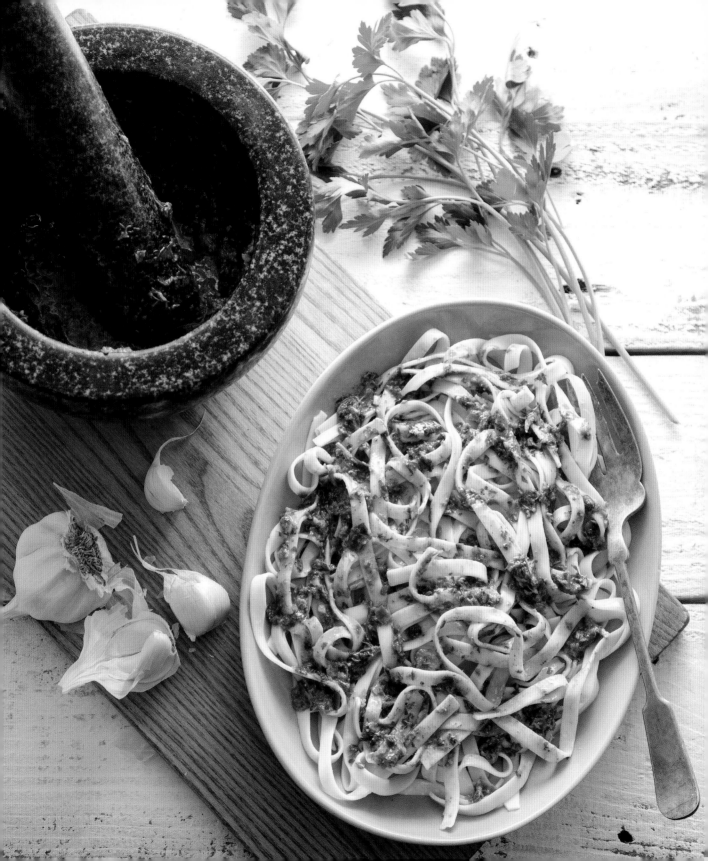

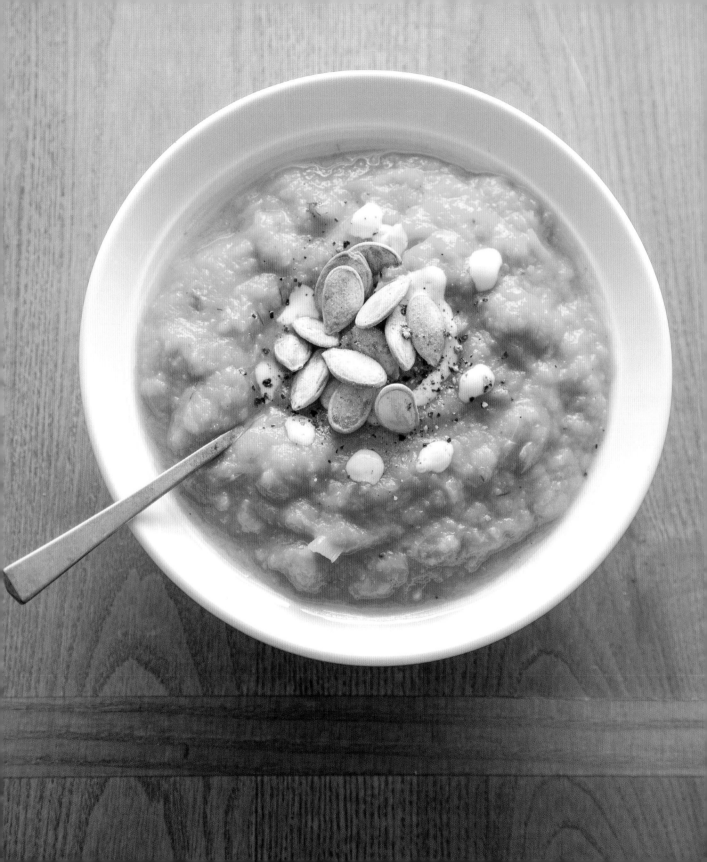

PUMPKIN SAFFRON SOUP

When it gets a little cooler outside and Pittas are loving their walks through the crisp air, Vatas are craving something warm. The creaminess of the coconut milk, the sweetness of the pumpkin and the sattvic qualities of the saffron combine to calm and clear any worrisome negative thoughts. Pumpkin is a cooling demulcent used topically for soft skin and internally for ulcers. Pumpkins have a diuretic action but are also high in potassium and sodium. The orange color indicates that pumpkin is also high in beta-carotene, useful for regeneration and rejuvenation—just what you need as you begin your cleanse.

YIELD: 4 servings

4 tbsp (60 g) ghee

1 leek, chopped

⅛ tsp saffron threads

2 tbsp (30 ml) apple cider vinegar

2 lb (910 g) pumpkin, peeled, seeded and chopped

2 carrots, chopped

4 cups (960 ml) vegetable broth or stock

⅛ tsp ground cinnamon

⅛ tsp ground nutmeg

¼ cup (60 ml) coconut milk

Salt and pepper, as desired

½ cup (70 g) toasted pumpkin seeds

In a large saucepan, melt the ghee. Add the leek and saffron and gently simmer, stirring occasionally, for about 5 minutes, or until tender. Add the vinegar, pumpkin, carrots, broth, cinnamon and nutmeg. Simmer for about 20 minutes, or until the pumpkin and carrots have softened.

Remove the pan from the heat and let it cool for 5 to 10 minutes. Transfer it to a blender and process until it's smooth and creamy. Return the soup to the saucepan and gently warm it.

Pour the soup into bowls and drizzle with coconut milk. Season with salt and pepper, sprinkle with toasted pumpkin seeds and serve immediately.

Dosha Adaptations

RECIPE WRITTEN FOR VATA.
PITTA: Omit the apple cider vinegar.
KAPHA: Add a pinch of red pepper flakes and omit the coconut milk.

ONE-POT SHAKSHUKA

As with all beans, chickpeas are *loaded* with fiber and protein. Chickpeas support healthy circulation and immunity, are rich in vitamins and are an excellent source of health-promoting fatty acids.

YIELD: 2 servings

1 tbsp (15 ml) extra-virgin olive oil or avocado oil

¼ white onion, diced

¼ red bell pepper, chopped

2 cloves garlic, minced

1 (15-oz [430-g]) can diced tomatoes

1½ tbsp (22 g) tomato paste

½ tbsp (7 g) coconut sugar or ½ tbsp (8 ml) maple syrup

Sea salt, as desired

1 tsp smoked or sweet paprika

½ tsp ground cumin

1 tsp chili powder

⅛ tsp ground cinnamon

1 (15-oz [430-g]) can chickpeas, rinsed and drained

2 cups (316 g) cooked basmati rice

Heat a large skillet over medium heat. Add the oil, onion, bell pepper and garlic. Sauté, stirring frequently, for 4 to 5 minutes, or until they're soft and fragrant. Add the tomatoes, tomato paste, coconut sugar, sea salt, paprika, cumin, chili powder and cinnamon. Stir to combine them. Bring it to a simmer over medium heat and cook for 2 to 3 minutes, stirring frequently. If you're okay with a chunkier texture, leave it as is. Or, scoop three-quarters of the sauce in the blender and process until it's smooth for a creamier result!

Add the chickpeas. Stir to combine them, and then reduce the heat to medium-low and simmer for 15 to 20 minutes to allow the flavors to develop and marry with the beans. Taste and adjust the seasonings as needed and serve over the rice.

Dosha Adaptations

RECIPE WRITTEN FOR VATA.

PITTA: Pittas should eat this meal sparingly. Take out the bell pepper, tomato paste and paprika. Add a cilantro garnish and a cooling yogurt dip.

KAPHA: No substitutions needed.

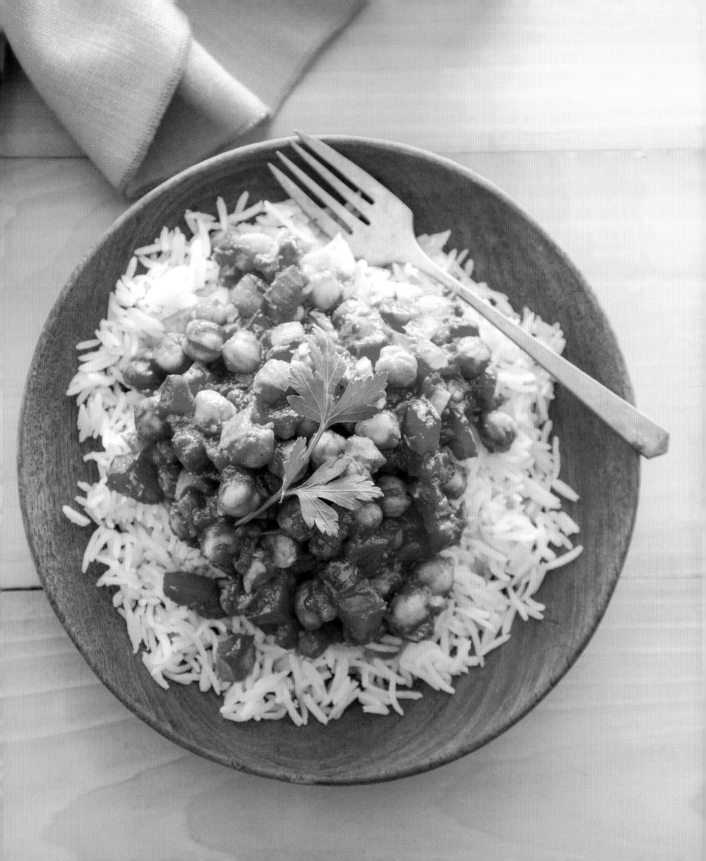

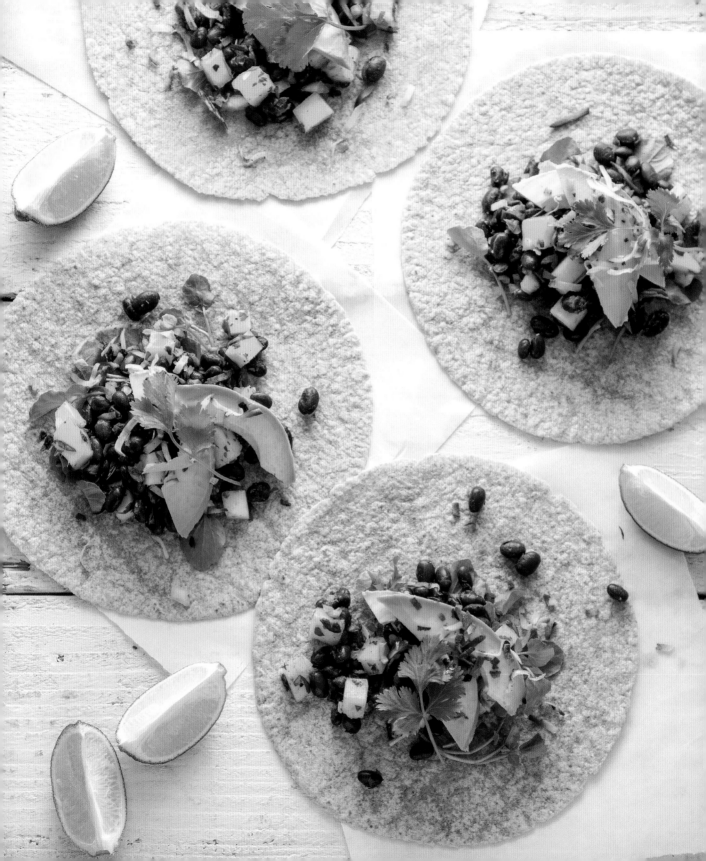

BLACK BEAN TACOS WITH MANGO SALSA

Satisfying and loaded with protein, beans are nature's remedy for strong food cravings. High in both soluble and insoluble fiber, the insoluble roughage stimulates bowel movements and helps to scrape the bowels. The fiber in beans also reduces cholesterol, all while increasing satisfaction. The hot spices kick-start the digestive system, stimulating your agni (digestive fire).

YIELD: 4 servings

1 (15-oz [430-g]) can black beans, drained and rinsed

1 large mango, cut into ¼" (6-mm) pieces

½ small onion, finely chopped

2 tbsp (30 ml) fresh lime juice

2 tsp (6 g) dosha-specific spice mix (page 32)

Pinch of asafetida (hing)

Salt and pepper, as desired

½ cup (20 g) chopped fresh cilantro

4 wheat tortillas, warmed

¼ cup (8 g) watercress

1 avocado, peeled, pitted and sliced

2 tbsp (10 g) toasted flaked coconut

Lime wedges, for serving

In a medium bowl, toss the beans, mango, onion, lime juice, dosha spice mix, asafetida, salt, pepper and cilantro.

Place each wheat tortilla on a serving plate. On top of each tortilla, place the watercress and top that with the bean and mango mixture. Add the avocado, sprinkle with the toasted coconut and serve with the lime wedges.

Dosha Adaptations

RECIPE WRITTEN FOR VATA.

PITTA: This is a perfect meal for Pittas. No substitutions needed.

KAPHA: Omit the toasted coconut and avocado and add ½ teaspoon of cayenne pepper to the salsa mix. Use corn tortillas.

WINTER FARRO SALAD

To make a great farro salad, we first cook it in apple cider along with a really good olive oil. The pistachios and cheese help make it a hearty, rich and warming protein-rich salad. Grains such as farro help build bone tissue and muscle and give bodily strength and endurance. Adequate quantities of grains are particularly important for those on a vegetarian diet.

YIELD: 2 servings

1 cup (200 g) uncooked farro

1 cup (240 ml) apple cider vinegar

2 tsp (10 g) kosher salt, plus more as needed

2 bay leaves

2 cups (480 ml) water, plus more as needed

½ cup (120 ml) extra-virgin olive oil

2 tbsp (30 ml) fresh lemon juice

½ cup (40 g) shaved Parmesan cheese

½ cup (60 g) chopped pistachio nuts

2 cups (40 g) arugula leaves

1 cup (24 g) basil or parsley leaves, torn

1 cup (24 g) mint leaves

1 cup (160 g) halved cherry or grape tomatoes

⅓ cup (40 g) thinly sliced radish

In a medium saucepan, add the farro, vinegar, salt, bay leaves and water and simmer for 30 minutes, or until the farro is tender and the liquid has evaporated. If all the liquid evaporates before the farro is done, add a little more water. Let the farro cool, and then discard the bay leaves.

In a salad bowl, whisk together the olive oil, lemon juice and a pinch of salt. Add the farro, Parmesan cheese and pistachio nuts and mix well. Just before serving, fold in the arugula, basil, mint, tomatoes, radish and salt to taste.

Dosha Adaptations

RECIPE WRITTEN FOR VATA.

PITTA: Omit the apple cider vinegar. Replace the tomatoes with red bell peppers.

KAPHA: Replace the tomatoes with red bell peppers and use goat cheese instead of Parmesan.

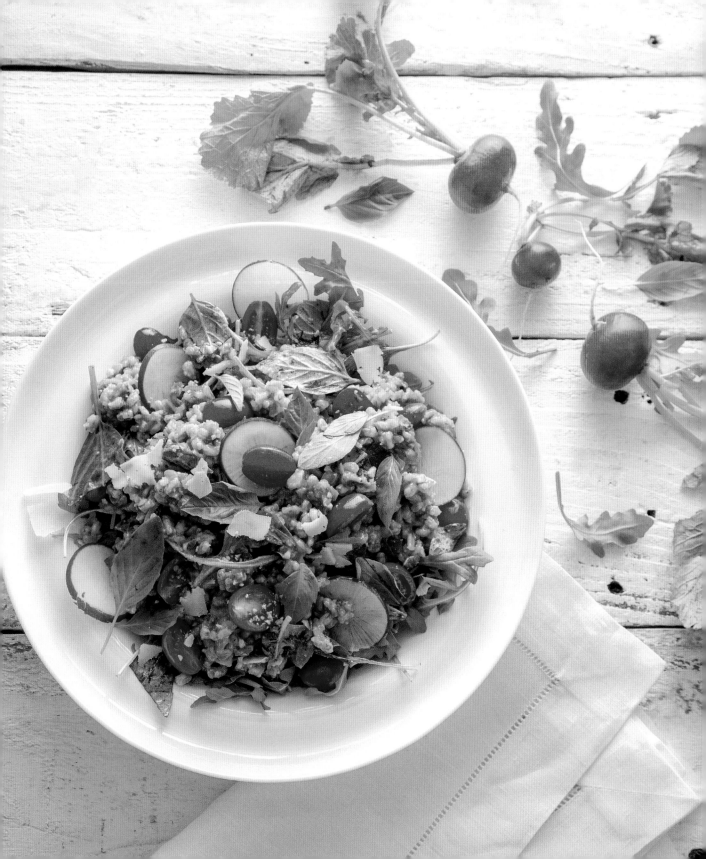

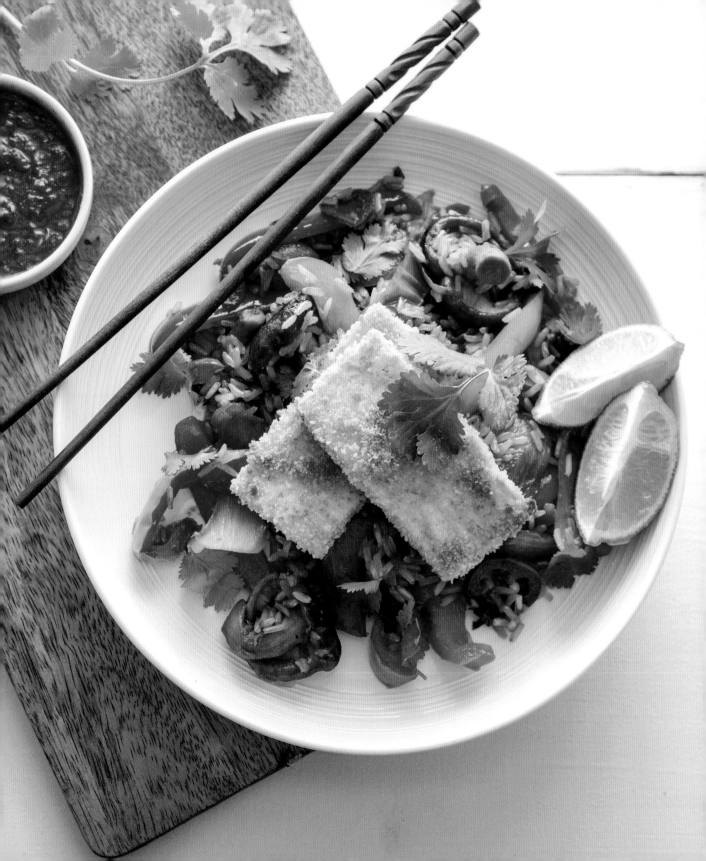

BAKED TOFU WITH GINGER RICE

Since most of us have to prepare dinner for ourselves, that means spending time in the kitchen before dinner is on the table. While shortcuts are nice, what we really want is to come home after work to a meal that takes as little prep time as possible. Try this crispy baked tofu and veggie stir-fry for a colorful low-prep meal that's packed with flavor. Ginger, with its pungent and sweet taste, warms the digestive system, increases agni (digestive fire) and helps in the secretion of digestive enzymes.

YIELD: 2 servings

1 cup (200 g) uncooked brown rice

1 lb (455 g) tofu

¼ cup (35 g) breadcrumbs

4 tsp (20 ml) extra-virgin olive oil, divided

1 egg

2 cloves garlic, crushed

2" (5-cm) piece ginger, peeled and grated

2 cups (320 g) vegetable stir-fry mix

2 tsp (10 ml) soy sauce

⅓ cup (15 g) chopped cilantro leaves, divided (optional)

Chili sauce, as desired

Lime wedges, for serving

Preheat the oven to 400°F (220°C). Cook the rice according to the package directions. Set it aside.

Drain the tofu and pat it with a paper towel to remove any excess moisture. Wrap it in a clean tea towel, place a heavy pan on top of it and leave the tofu to dry out until it's needed.

In a shallow bowl, mix the breadcrumbs with 2 teaspoons (10 ml) of the oil. In a separate shallow bowl, beat the egg. Cut the tofu into 16 pieces and dip each piece in the egg, and then coat them with the breadcrumbs. Transfer the tofu to a nonstick baking tray and bake for 20 minutes, or until browned but not burned.

In a wok, heat the remaining 2 teaspoons (10 ml) oil over medium heat. Add the garlic, ginger and vegetable mix and stir-fry for 2 minutes. Add the rice and stir-fry for 3 minutes, or until it's piping hot. Stir in the soy sauce and half the cilantro (if using), and then serve with the tofu, a drizzle of chili sauce, the remaining cilantro and lime wedges for squeezing.

Dosha Adaptations

RECIPE WRITTEN FOR VATA.

PITTA: Remove the chili sauce.

KAPHA: No substitutions needed.

JICAMA SALAD
WITH MINTY TAHINI SAUCE

Raw veggies aren't always the best option for good digestion. In fact, they can slow digestive fire (agni) for all doshas. However, these veggies, including jicama, are actually some of the best veggies to consume raw as they have high water content. Jicama is also high in fiber, and the particular fiber of this tuber feeds the good-gut microbes in your digestive system. This meal is light, crunchy, astringent yet satisfying and distinctly flavorful for an evening meal.

YIELD: 2 servings

3 tbsp (20 g) raw pumpkin seeds

1 tsp sesame seeds

2 tbsp (30 ml) freshly squeezed lime juice

1 tbsp (3 g) finely chopped fresh basil

Pinch of red pepper flakes

Salt and pepper, as desired

⅓ cup (75 g) tahini

1 clove garlic, minced

1 handful fresh mint leaves, plus more as needed

2 medium carrots, peeled and julienned

1 cup (140 g) diced English cucumber

1 medium jicama, peeled and sliced

In a small bowl, combine the pumpkin seeds, sesame seeds, lime juice, basil, red pepper flakes, salt and pepper. Add the contents of the bowl to a blender along with the tahini, garlic and mint. Process until it's smooth and creamy.

In a large bowl, mix the carrots, cucumber and jicama. Pour the sauce over the vegetables and toss well to coat them. Serve with more shredded mint leaves, as desired.

Dosha Adaptations

RECIPE WRITTEN FOR VATA.
PITTA: This is a perfect meal for Pittas. No substitutions needed.
KAPHA: This is a great meal for Kaphas, but use soy yogurt instead of tahini.

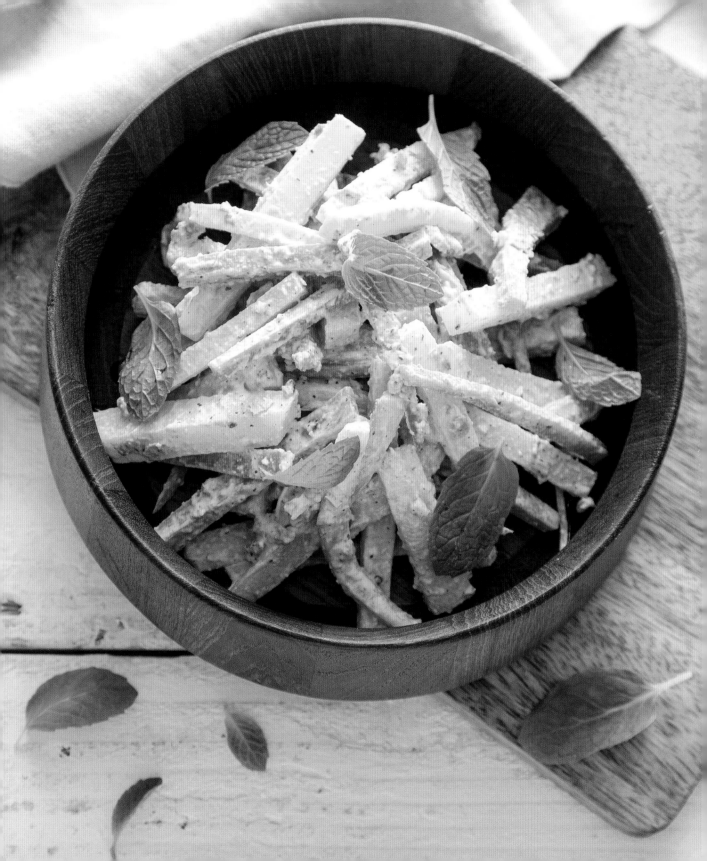

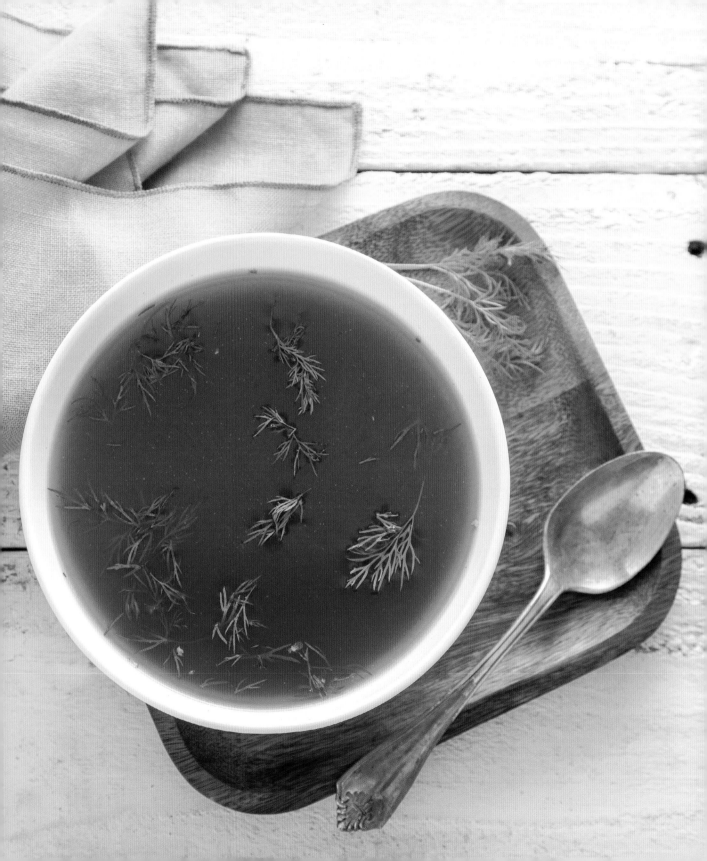

FENUGREEK AND DILL WEIGHT-LOSS SOUP

Fenugreek reduces inflammation and is a highly effective herb when it comes to imbalances of Vata and Kapha. Not only is it warming, but it also has a sweet taste and a nourishing, unctuous quality, which creates a strong grounding effect in the body. It also strengthens the central digestive fire as the seeds keep the plasma and blood healthy. When we combine fenugreek with dill, the health benefits double with this soup's ability to boost digestive health as well as provide relief from insomnia, hiccups, diarrhea, dysentery, menstrual disorders, respiratory disorders and cancer.

YIELD: 2 servings

4 cups (960 ml) vegetable broth or stock

1 tsp ground fenugreek

1 tsp ground ginger

1 tsp dill

1 tsp dosha-specific spice mix (page 32)

Pepper, as desired

½ tsp ghee

In a soup pot, bring the vegetable broth to a boil over medium heat. Stir in the fenugreek, ginger, dill, dosha spice mix and pepper. Reduce the heat and simmer for 15 minutes. Serve in a soup bowl along with the ghee and more pepper to taste.

Dosha Adaptations

RECIPE WRITTEN FOR VATA.
PITTA: No substitutions needed.
KAPHA: This is a great soup for Kaphas.

ZUCCHINI NOODLES WITH PESTO

There are a lot of rejuvenating ingredients in this dish that are designed to balance, cool and calm. The cilantro, almonds and mint turn this dish into a healthy and energizing meal full of antioxidants and phytonutrients. The menthol in the mint helps the digestive process along by acting on the smooth muscles of the stomach. The aroma of mint activates the salivary glands as well as the glands that produce digestive enzymes. As a result, our digestion improves.

YIELD: 2 servings

5–6 medium zucchinis, trimmed

¾ tsp salt, divided

1 ripe avocado, peeled and pitted

1 cup (20 g) packed fresh cilantro leaves

¼ cup (35 g) unsalted almonds

2 tbsp (30 ml) lemon juice

¼ tsp ground pepper

5 tbsp (75 ml) extra-virgin olive oil, divided

3 cloves garlic, minced

Mint leaves, as desired

Using a spiral vegetable slicer or a vegetable peeler, cut the zucchini lengthwise into long, thin strands or strips. Stop when you reach the seeds in the middle. (Seeds make the zucchini noodles fall apart.) Place the zucchini noodles in a colander and toss them with ½ teaspoon of the salt. Let the noodles drain for 15 to 30 minutes, and then gently squeeze them to remove any excess water.

In a food processor, combine the avocado, cilantro, almonds, lemon juice, pepper and remaining ¼ teaspoon of salt. Pulse until it's finely chopped. Add 4 tablespoons (60 ml) of the olive oil and process until it's smooth. Set it aside.

In a large skillet, heat the remaining 1 tablespoon (15 ml) of olive oil over medium-high heat. Add the garlic and cook, stirring, for 30 seconds. Add the zucchini noodles and mint. Gently toss them for 3 minutes, or until hot. Transfer the zucchini noodles to a serving bowl, add the avocado-cilantro "pesto" and gently toss to combine them.

Dosha Adaptations

RECIPE WRITTEN FOR VATA.
PITTA: No substitutions needed.
KAPHA: Use sunflower oil instead of olive oil.

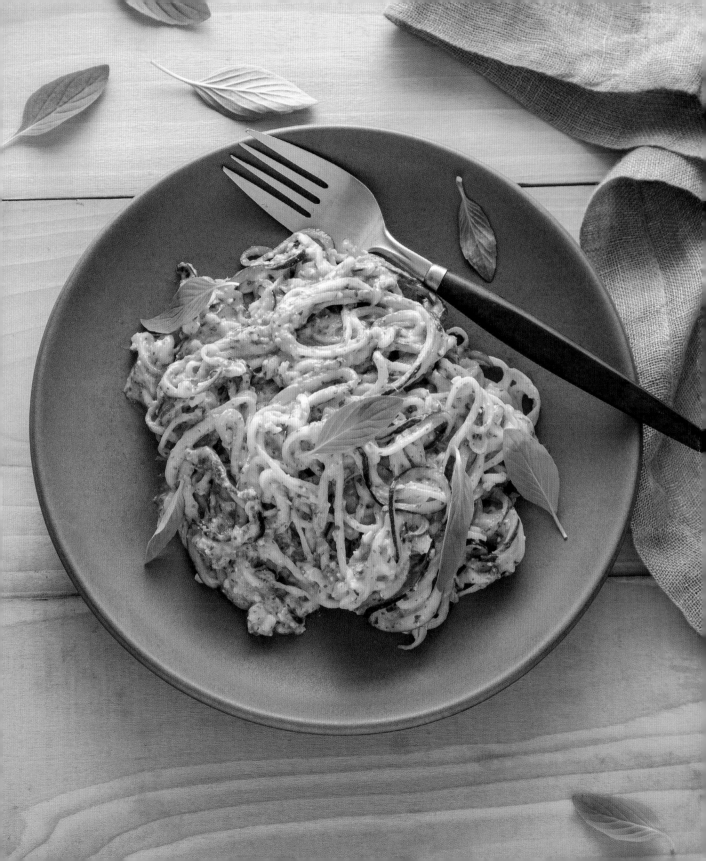

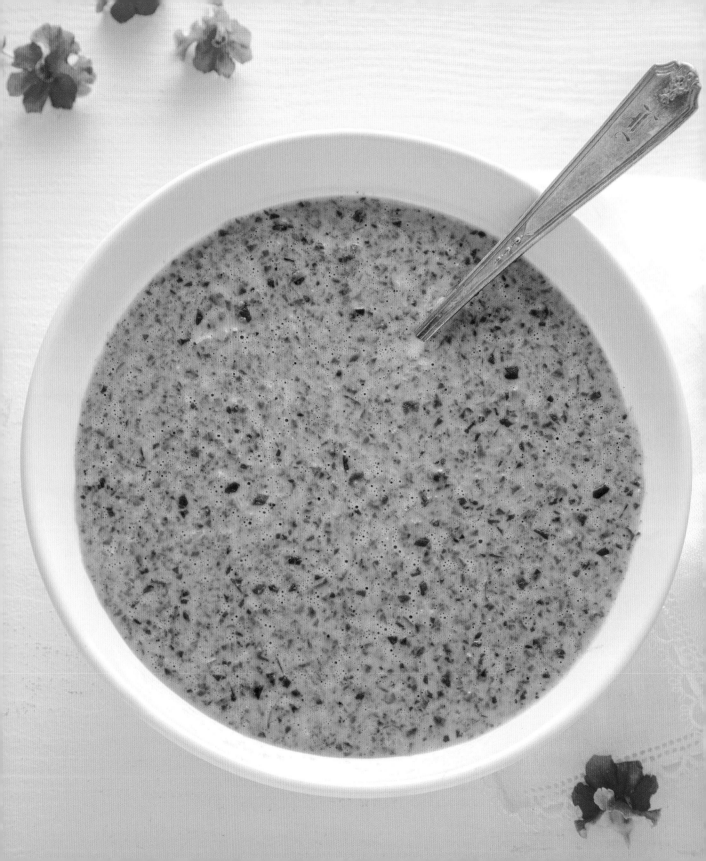

COOLING COCONUT CURRY SOUP

This curry is as flavorful as it is easy to make. Prepared with a predominantly sweet, post-digestive effect that balances Vata and Pitta, this is a natural stress-buster that is not only delicious but healing.

YIELD: 2 servings

1 tbsp (14 g) coconut oil

2 cloves garlic, minced

1 shallot, diced

½ tbsp (4 g) minced ginger

½ tbsp (4 g) curry powder, plus more to taste

4 oz (115 g) frozen spinach, slightly thawed

1⅓ cups (320 ml) unsweetened light coconut milk

½ tbsp (7 g) coconut sugar, plus more to taste

Sea salt, as desired

1–2 tbsp (10–20 g) cornstarch or arrowroot starch

Cooked basmati rice, as desired

Heat a large skillet or pot over medium heat. Add the oil, garlic, shallot and ginger. Cook, stirring frequently, for 3 to 4 minutes, or until they're softened and slightly browned. Add the curry and spinach and cook for 3 to 4 minutes, stirring occasionally. Add the coconut milk, coconut sugar and salt. Simmer for 4 minutes. Add the cornstarch and stir. Reduce the heat to low and cook for 5 to 10 minutes, or until it's slightly thickened. Serve with rice, if desired.

Dosha Adaptations

RECIPE WRITTEN FOR VATA.

PITTA: Add toasted coconut as a garnish.

KAPHA: No substitutions needed.

AMAZING MUSHROOM SOUP

Did you know that the heavy earthiness of mushrooms are excellent for any kind of insomnia? Add some ginger and turmeric and you've got a powerful one-two anti-inflammatory punch!

YIELD: 4 servings

1 tbsp (15 g) ghee

1 onion, chopped

1 cup (60 g) chopped mushrooms

3½ cups (840 ml) vegetable broth or stock

1 tsp grated ginger

Pinch of ground coriander

1 tsp ground turmeric

Salt and pepper, as desired

In a large saucepan, heat the ghee and cook the onion for about 5 minutes, or until it's translucent. Add the mushrooms and sauté for 2 minutes. Add the broth, bring it to a boil and simmer for 5 minutes. Add the ginger, coriander, turmeric, salt and pepper and cook for 7 to 8 minutes, or until the soup is fragrant. Season to taste and enjoy!

Dosha Adaptations
RECIPE WRITTEN FOR VATA.
PITTA: No substitutions needed.
KAPHA: No substitutions needed.

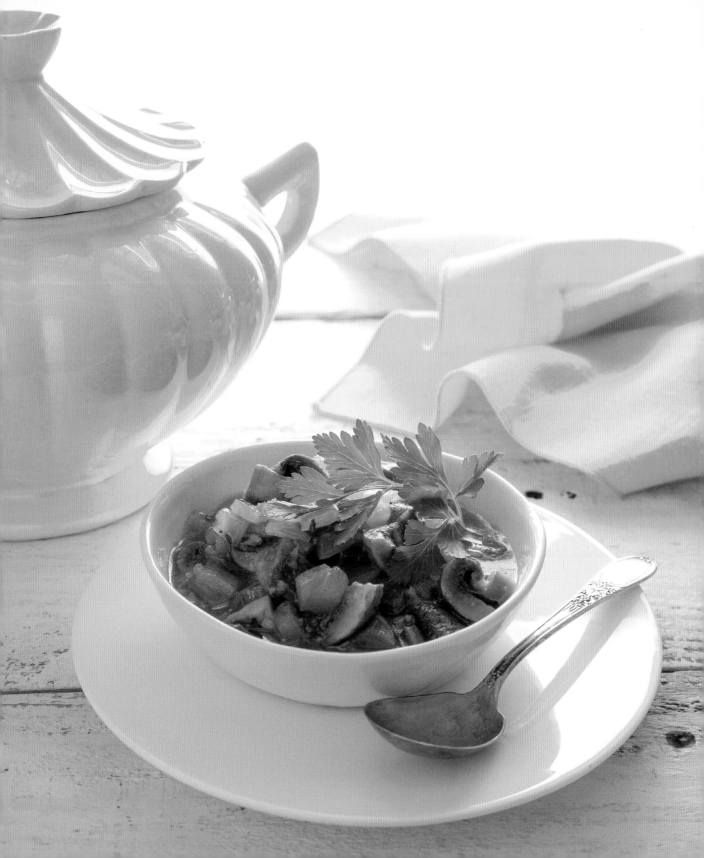

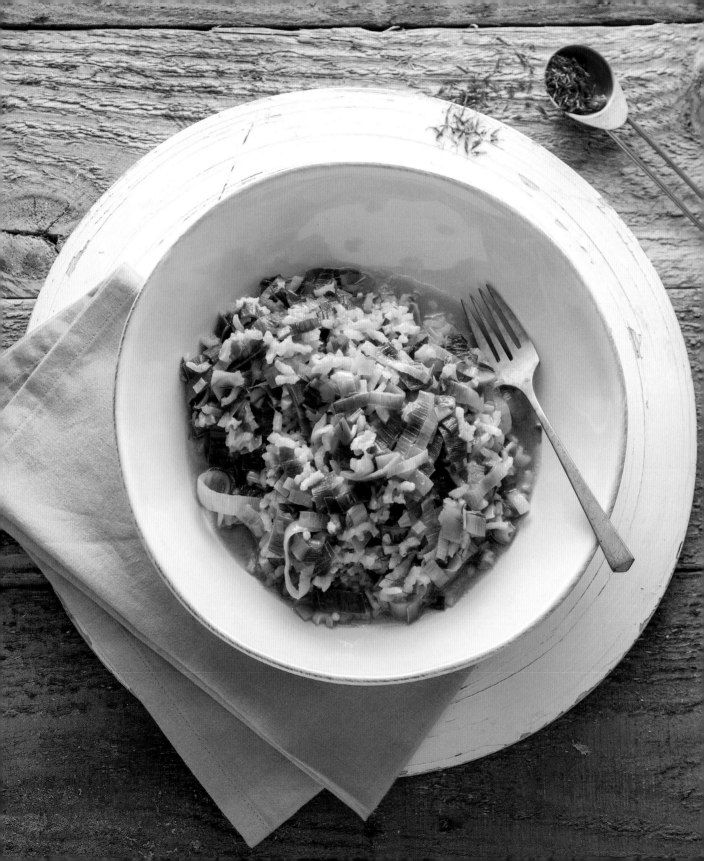

SAFFRON LENTIL RISOTTO

Saffron is famous for its medicinal, coloring and flavoring properties. Valued all over the world, especially by culinary and medical experts, its snigdha (oily) and laghu (light) properties, along with its bitter taste, pacifies all doshas. Saffron also has a unique vipaka (post-digestive process) that helps assimilate nutrition, and when cleansing, we need all the nutritional help we can get.

YIELD: 2 servings

3 cups (720 ml) vegetable broth
1½ tbsp (22 g) ghee, divided
2 leek stalks, washed and sliced
⅔ cup (130 g) uncooked risotto rice
½ cup (120 ml) white wine, at room temperature
Pinch of Italian saffron
Salt and pepper, as desired
Chopped parsley, for garnishing

In a medium pot, bring the broth to a gentle boil.

In a large pot, melt 1 tablespoon (15 g) of the ghee. Add the leeks and roast over medium heat for 5 minutes, or until they're tender. Add the rice and toast it with the leek for 2 to 3 minutes, or until slightly browned. Add the wine and let it evaporate, 1 to 2 minutes, while stirring constantly.

Add the vegetable broth, one ladle at a time, while stirring frequently. Ensure that both the risotto and the broth are kept simmering. Retain 1 ladle of the broth. Cook, covered, for 10 minutes.

Dissolve the saffron in the remaining ladle of broth and then add it to the rice. Cook, covered, for 5 to 8 minutes, or until the rice is soft and there's no excess liquid left in the pot. Stir in the remaining ½ tablespoon (7 g) ghee, season with salt and pepper and let the risotto rest for 1 minute. Serve sprinkled with the chopped parsley.

Dosha Adaptations
RECIPE WRITTEN FOR VATA.
PITTA: Serve with chopped cilantro instead of parsley.
KAPHA: Garnish with chopped basil instead of parsley.

PUMPKIN PASTA

Pumpkin is a cooling demulcent used topically for softer skin and internally for ulcers. Pumpkins have a diuretic action but are also high in potassium and sodium. The orange color indicates that pumpkin is high in beta-carotene, useful for regeneration. Pumpkins also have a sedative and laxative effect—all designed to help that sluggish digestion as we cleanse.

YIELD: 4 servings

1 (16-oz [455-g]) box wheat penne

2 tbsp (30 g) ghee, divided

4 cloves garlic, chopped

1 medium onion, finely chopped

1 bay leaf

4–6 sage sprigs, cut into chiffonade, plus more for garnishing

½ cup (120 ml) dry white wine, at room temperature

2 cups (480 ml) vegetable broth or stock

1 cup (245 g) canned pumpkin

½ cup (120 ml) almond cream

⅛ tsp ground cinnamon

½ tsp ground nutmeg

Salt and pepper, as desired

Cook the pasta until al dente according to the package directions. Set it aside.

Heat a large skillet over medium-high heat. Add 1 tablespoon (15 g) of the ghee and sauté the garlic and onion for 3 to 5 minutes, or until the onion is tender. Add the bay leaf, sage and wine to the pan. Cook for 2 minutes, or until the wine is reduced by half. Add the broth and pumpkin and stir to combine them. Keep stirring until the sauce begins to boil. Stir in the almond cream. Season with the cinnamon, nutmeg, salt and pepper. Simmer for 5 to 10 minutes, or until the sauce thickens.

Return the pasta to the pot you cooked it in. Remove the bay leaf from the sauce and pour it over the pasta. Toss it over low heat for 1 minute. Garnish with lots of sage leaves and serve.

Dosha Adaptations

RECIPE WRITTEN FOR VATA.
PITTA: Remove the nutmeg and garlic and add 1 teaspoon of cilantro or mint instead.
KAPHA: Switch out the wheat pasta for a corn pasta (look for this in the gluten-free aisle of your grocery store).

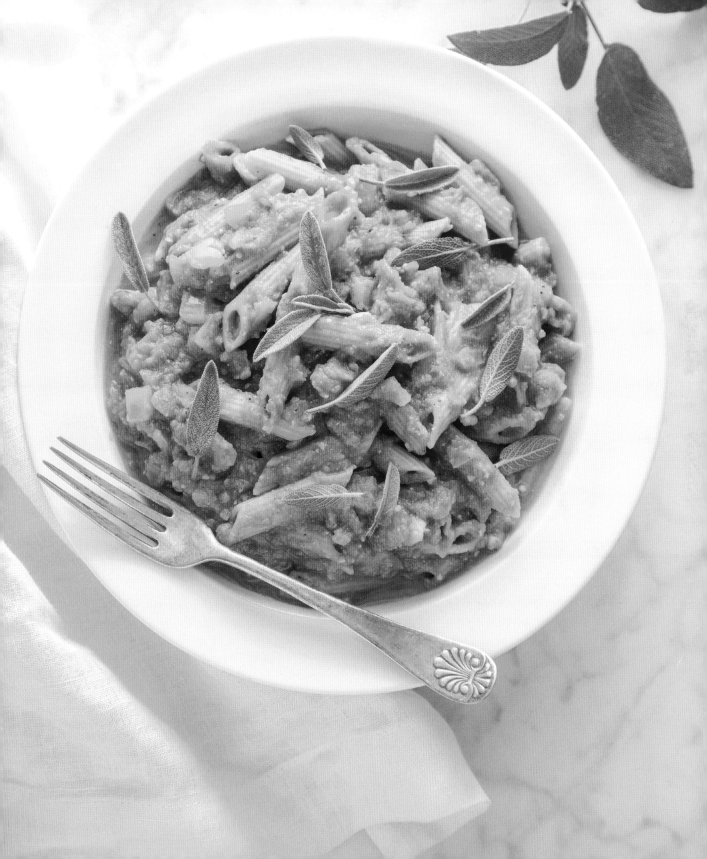

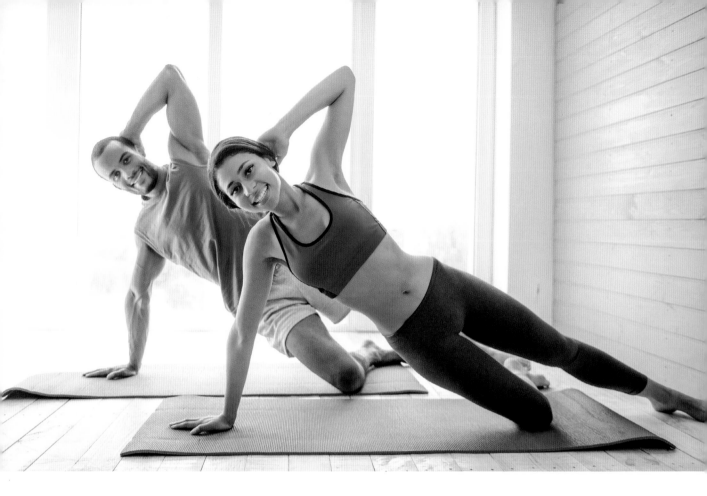

SELF-CARE

Self-care is not indulgent or selfish; it is necessary to feel truly healthy and vital. Daily self-care helps cultivate habits that will suffuse all aspects of your life. When we practice simple acts of self-care through yoga, meditation and pranayama (breathwork), we are allowing ourselves to feel deeply nourished.

Follow these practices in a quiet, grounded and systematic way. Allow yourself the time to practice, and tell yourself that you have nowhere else to go, nothing else to do. This is your time to take care of yourself.

Yoga Sequence for Strength and Flexibility

This yoga practice will bring balance to your overstimulated mind and stressed body. It is designed to build your core while maintaining flexibility. The balance between flexibility and strength will benefit you immensely as you start your cleanse. Work with the breath, and hold the poses just a little longer than is comfortable. Remaining still and calm will be your challenge and your reward. Don't worry if what you do doesn't look like the images yet. This is your practice, and consistent effort is more valuable to your body than cramming yourself into a pose just so you can look like the model. The entire sequence should take about 24 to 26 minutes. If you would like to join me with your yoga or meditation, go to www.theholistichighway.com/bookspecial and type in the password "Ayurveda." Here you'll find videos and audio to accompany the book, and we can do this together.

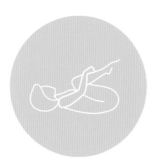

Lovin' Your Back (2 minutes)

1. Lie on your back. Bend your knees and draw them in toward your chest. Clasp your hands around your knees or shins.

2. Rock slowly and gently from side to side, massaging your lower back.

3. Keep the knees together and circle them first in one direction and then the other as you enjoy the opening and relaxing of your lower back area.

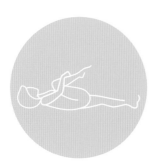

Wind Releasing Time (1 minute)

1. Stay lying on your back. Keep your right leg bent into your chest and extend your left leg straight out to the floor. Keep your hands clasped around the knee or shin of the right leg.

2. Breathe slowly and deeply as you feel your colon being massaged. This will improve digestion and elimination.

3. Exhale—releasing the right leg straight out on the floor. Inhale—draw the left leg toward the chest, massaging the colon again (take 3 to 5 deep breaths). Exhale—release the left leg to the ground.

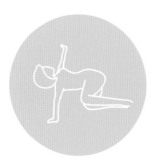

Twist It Up (2 minutes)

1. Stay lying on your back with your knees bent and feet flat on the floor.

2. Make a T-position of your body with your arms stretched out to the side.

3. Inhale. And as you exhale, take the bent knees over to the floor on your right side, creating an elongated twist through your spine.

4. Turn your head to look in the opposite direction of the twist. Allow yourself between 3 to 5 deep breaths.

5. Inhale—bringing your knees back to the starting position. Exhale—and repeat on the other side.

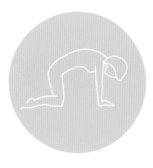

Cat Stretch (1 minute)

1. Come up onto your hands and knees. Place your shoulders directly above your wrists and your hips directly over your knees. Spread your fingers open like a fan and press the entire surface of your hands into the floor.

2. Inhale, drawing your tailbone toward the sky and dipping your abdomen toward the earth. Continue this movement until your chest and gaze are moving upwards.

3. Exhale, drawing your tailbone back toward the ground as you lift your navel up toward the ceiling. Bring your chin toward your chest to lengthen the back of your neck. Repeat 5 times.

Child Pose (2 minutes)

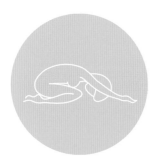

1. Press your bottom back to sit on your heels and lay your chest on your legs, resting your forehead on the ground. If your bottom does not quite reach your heels, just place a folded blanket on your thighs, so you can enjoy the pose.

2. Place your arms and hands on the floor with your palms facing up and elbows slightly bent. Breathe deeply into the belly about 10 times.

Tree Balance (1 minute)

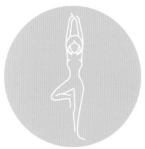

1. Stand with your weight equally distributed between both feet. Begin to shift your body weight toward the right foot. Place the ball of your left foot to the right ankle or on the side of the right calf or inner thigh (not beside the right knee). Keep your pelvis square to the front of the room.

2. Bring your hands together in front of your heart or above your head. Breathe comfortably as you balance on one leg. Smile and stay as long as you can. Repeat on the other side.

Triangle (2 minutes)

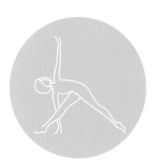

1. Stand with both feet together. Move the left leg approximately 3 to 4 feet (0.9 to 1.2 m) to the side and place the left foot on a forward angle of about 45 degrees.

2. Inhale—raise both arms up to shoulder height. Exhale—shift the weight of your pelvis toward the left as you reach to the side with the torso and right arm (keeping both sides of the torso long and even).

3. Place the right hand on the right leg without collapsing your body weight into it. Look up toward the left hand. Breathe here for 5 full breaths.

4. Inhale—to press into your feet, engage your core and return upright. Exhale—lower your hands to your hips. Inhale—step the left foot forward beside the right foot. Repeat on the second side.

Wind Down Waterfall (3–5 minutes)

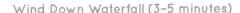

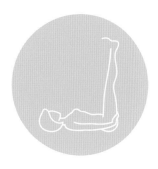

1. Sit sideways with your right hip against the wall.

2. Use the support of your hands to gently roll yourself onto your back with your legs up against the wall. Your sitting bones should touch the wall. Relax your entire body as your legs stay extended up the wall in alignment with your hips. Your arms are comfortably out to the side, palms up.

3. To come out of this restorative pose, bend your knees and push your feet against the wall to slide the body away from the wall. Then turn to your right side and rest here for a few minutes. Use your arms to push yourself up to sitting.

Save-It Savasana (10 minutes)

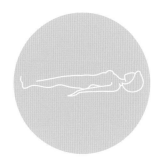

1. Lie down comfortably on your back with your legs extended. Cover yourself with a blanket if you are apt to get cold.

2. Pull the shoulders down and back as you lengthen your arms along your side, palms up. Lengthen your neck. Inhale deeply, exhale and allow your whole body to relax.

3. Systematically relax each part of your body beginning with your feet. Relax your toes, then ankles, then calves, knees and hips, all while moving your awareness up through your body, consciously relaxing any stress or tight spots along the way. Keep your breath deep and natural and allow yourself to surrender into the stillness of this pose.

4. After about 10 minutes, slowly deepen your breath, wiggle your fingers and toes, bring some movement back into your body by stretching in any way that feels good to you.

5. Roll onto your right side, stay there for a couple of moments and then use your hands to push yourself into an upright seated position.

After doing these poses, take a few minutes to come back and ask yourself how you are feeling. How has this practice changed you? Take a moment to acknowledge your efforts and your commitment to your daily practice. Bring your hands to your heart center in a prayer position and allow yourself to appreciate whatever it is that brings joy into your life.

Loving-Kindness Meditation

If you would like to join me with your yoga or meditation, go to www.theholistichighway.com/bookspecial and type in the password "Ayurveda." Here you'll find videos and audio to accompany the book, and we can do this together.

Say to yourself:

May I be happy.
May I be safe.
May I be healthy and free from suffering.
May I be at peace—just as I am now.

Now think of someone you love—someone who has been there for you, and as you think of them—repeat in your mind:

May you be happy.
May you be safe.
May you be healthy and free from suffering.
May you be at peace—just as you are now.

Now think of the whole world and everyone and everything in it, and repeat in your mind:

May all beings be happy.
May all beings be safe.
May all beings be healthy and free from suffering.
May all beings be at peace—just as they are now.

Pranayama: Alternate Nostril Breathing

To reduce stress in your body, there is a powerful practice of breathing called alternate nostril breathing, or *nadi shodhana*. This form of breathing can neutralize the cortisol in your body that stimulates the stress response. Through a daily practice of alternate nostril breathing, you will see better sleep, more focus, better memory and a clearer mind.

1. Sit on a chair or on the floor in a comfortable position with your spine lengthened and your shoulders down and relaxed. Relax your face and jaw and concentrate on a slow and steady breathing pattern.

2. Place your left hand on your right knee and rest your right thumb on your right nostril and your right ring finger gently resting on your left nostril. Take a slow, deep breath.

3. Close off your right nostril with your thumb and exhale slowly through your left nostril. After you have gently breathed in again through the left nostril, close the left nostril with your ring finger and exhale through the right nostril.

4. Now inhale through your right nostril. At the top of the breath, close the right nostril by pressing the thumb to close it and exhale out through the left nostril. Practice 10 rounds of this breath.

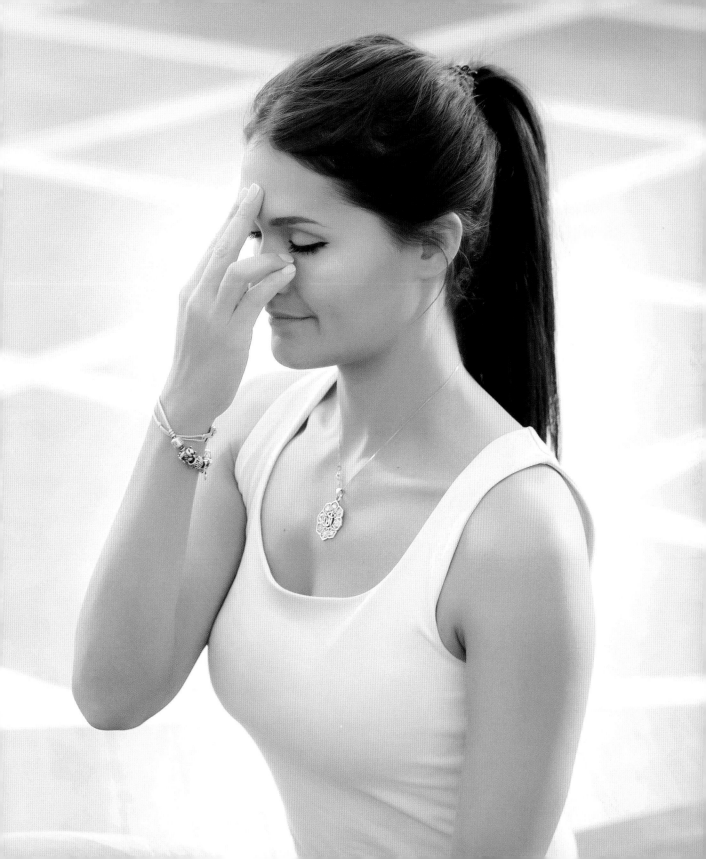

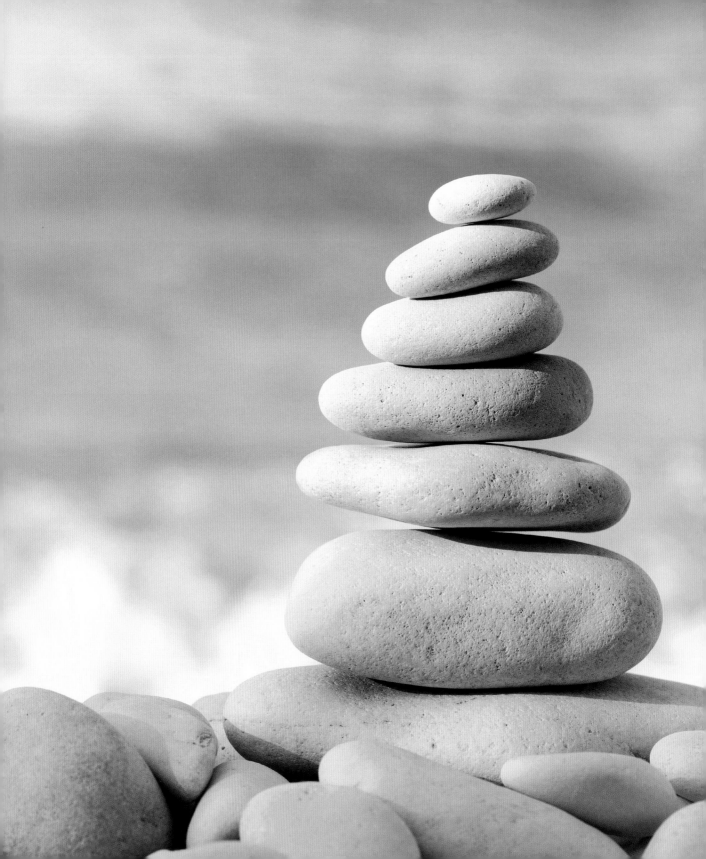

Chapter 3

PHASE 2
DAYS 12 TO 19

"The doctor of the future will give no medication, but will interest his patients in the care of the human frame, diet and in the cause and prevention of disease." —Thomas Edison

ACTIVE CLEANSE: THE HEART OF THE PROGRAM

This is the heart of the cleanse. During this time, you will be eating a mono-diet of very simple, cleansing foods, such as Kitchari (page 132). The diet is substantive enough that you can maintain your essential responsibilities, but it simultaneously resets the digestive system, supports the elimination of toxins and balances Vata, Pitta and Kapha.

This is the transformative part of the cleanse and that means losing unwanted fat, getting that glow back, recharging your metabolism, balancing your hormones, ditching the belly bloat and losing the toxins that keep you feeling sluggish. You will feel happier and more alert as you ignite the fire within you. You will start filling your energy tank all the way.

Eat Clean

Did you know that 95 percent of your serotonin (the happy hormone) is manufactured in your digestive system? And did you know 80 percent of your immune system is also manufactured in your digestive system? During the active cleanse, you are strengthening your digestive system, the gateway to your health. You will boost your immune system, lose weight with ease, feel less bloated, uncover hidden food allergies and most of all, digest with ease.

DAILY ROUTINE

As you follow your daily routine, take a look at the day-by-day suggestions for your active cleanse during days 12 to 19.

Phase 2 Daily Routine

	VATA	PITTA	KAPHA
Wake Up	½ hour before sunrise (in spring and summer in the Northern Hemisphere, feel free to get up just before sunrise)	1 hour before sunrise (in spring and summer in the Northern Hemisphere, feel free to get up ½ hour before sunrise)	1½ hours before sunrise (in spring and summer in the Northern Hemisphere, feel free to get up 45 minutes before sunrise)
Drink	Vata Cleansing Tea (page 31)	Pitta Cooling Tea (page 31)	Kapha Stimulating Tea (page 31)
Nose	Add a few drops of sesame oil or nasya oil into both nostrils (see page 35).		
Exercise	Follow Yoga Sequence (page 137).		
Abhyanga (oil massage)	Sesame Oil	Coconut Oil	Sesame or Mustard Oil
Facial Wash & Serum	Vata Facial Wash (page 120)	Pitta Facial Wash (page 120)	Kapha Facial Wash (page 120)
Meditation Practice	Spend 15 minutes minimum on your daily spiritual practice. See journal suggestions.		
Breakfast	Vata Seasonal Cleanse Breakfast (pages 124–131)	Pitta Seasonal Cleanse Breakfast (pages 124–131)	Kapha Seasonal Cleanse Breakfast (pages 124–131)
Mid-Morning	Take 2 trikatu tablets (see page 37). Vata Cleansing Tea (page 31)	Pitta Cooling Tea (page 31)	Take 2 trikatu tablets (see page 37). Kapha Stimulating Tea (page 31)
Lunch (12 p.m. to 2 p.m.)	Kitchari (page 132) with Vata Spice (page 32) Hot water to drink Rest after lunch.	Kitchari (page 132) with Pitta Spice (page 32) Room temperature water to drink Take a short walk in nature after lunch.	Kitchari (page 132) with Kapha Spice (page 32) Hot water to drink Take a brisk walk after lunch.

	VATA	PITTA	KAPHA
Mid-Afternoon	Vata Cleansing Tea (page 31) You can take a nap or rest.	Pitta Cooling Tea (page 31) Take a break.	Kapha Stimulating Tea (page 31) Take some quick breaths or try kapalabhati breathing (page 143).
Dinner (5:30 p.m. to 7:30 p.m.)	Kitchari (page 132) Drink hot water.	Kitchari (page 132) Drink room temperature water.	Kitchari (page 132) Drink hot water.
Sunset	Some gentle stretching or yoga sequence	A cooling walk or yoga sequence	A brisk walk or yoga sequence
Journal Practice	See journal suggestions.		
Nighttime	Take 2 triphala tablets or 1 tsp triphala powder in warm water. If you experience constipation, you can take up to 4 tablets or 2 tsp (10 g) triphala powder in warm water.	Take 2 triphala tablets or 1 tsp triphala powder in warm water. If you experience any diarrhea or loose stools, reduce the triphala to 1 tablet or ½ tsp powder in warm water.	Take 2 triphala tablets or 1 tsp triphala powder in water. Kaphas do not normally experience constipation or diarrhea.
Massage	Follow the instructions for abhyanga (page 137) and massage the soles of your feet with sesame oil before bed.	Follow the instructions for abhyanga (page 137) and massage the soles of your feet with coconut oil before bed.	Follow the instructions for abhyanga (page 137) and massage the soles of your feet with sesame oil or mustard oil before bed.
Essential Oil	Spray your bedroom with your Vata aromatic mister (page 121).	Spray your bedroom with your Pitta aromatic mister (page 121).	Spray your bedroom with your Kapha aromatic mister (page 121).
Mantra Before Sleep	I am no longer fearful and have faith that I am safe and confident in everything that I do.	I am just one small part of the world and have lots of compassion for others. Each person is important.	I practice nonattachment and can easily let go of things that are no longer needed.

DAY 12

It is best not to eat until the majority of the laxative effect of the castor oil from Day 11 has worn off. One of three things will happen:

1. You wake up with a strong urge to eliminate, you have several bowel movements and then feel hungry. If this is the case, go ahead and eat your dosha breakfast followed by Kitchari (page 132) for lunch and dinner. You are fine to move ahead.

2. You wake up with the urge to eliminate and at lunch time you are still eliminating. You do not feel hungry and in fact feel a little nauseated and weak. If this is the case, drink some warm water with honey, rest and then have Kitchari (page 132) for your evening meal.

3. You wake up and nothing has happened. In fact, you got all psyched up . . . for nothing! This does happen to about 10 percent of people. Do not start the Kitchari (page 132) yet, but take your castor oil again tonight and repeat the procedure.

Journal Entry: What brings you joy and allows you to feel confident in the world?

DAY 13

It's Kitchari (page 132) for all meals except breakfast. Enjoy the breakfast that is right for your dosha. And just slow down! Drink three to four glasses of plain hot water per day. This is very important to flush out the system.

Journal Entry: Some of the things that make me happy are . . .

DAY 14

Keep on keeping on! How about adding a chutney to your Kitchari (page 132) in case you are getting a wee bit bored of Kitchari? If you are a Vata or Kapha, add the Sesame Seed Chutney (page 135) and if you are a Pitta, add the Fresh Coriander Chutney (page 135).

Journal Entry: What do you love about the season you are in? Can you bring some of that season indoors?

DAY 15

Kitchari for lunch and dinner when hungry. Get creative with seasonal greens (kale, chard, spinach and collards).

Journal Entry: Think about all the joy and angst you had as a child. Can you remember what you wanted to be when you grew up? How has the child in you changed through the years? What parts of that child would you like to embrace and what parts would you like to let go?

DAY 16

Kitchari for all meals when hungry. You can have it for breakfast too if you like, but I find most people prefer their specific dosha breakfast. You are doing great! Put on your sneakers or yoga clothes because exercise is vital for digestion. Get moving! When you move your body, you move your prana (the vital energy in your body), and this is key for your digestion. Even if you can only manage 12 to 15 minutes per day, get your heart pumping and your digestion will improve. Plus, you will release key endorphins that make you feel happy and less hungry.

Journal Entry: As a kid, how did you like to move? Did you cartwheel, roll down hills or did you just love to run? Capture that feeling and write about it.

DAY 17

Are you taking the time to enjoy your breakfast? Has it become important to you now? Are you adding your ghee? It's a great way to improve digestion and overall health. Ghee has been around for centuries, and by adding this high-quality prebiotic to your life, you will assimilate your nutrients better, have clearer skin, get better sleep and enjoy decreased inflammation.

Journal Entry: What did you used to do that had you so engrossed that you forgot all sense of time? Maybe you danced, drew, took pictures or marveled at the clouds. When was the last time you felt that way? Can you feel that way again? What would it take?

DAY 18

You're in a groove now. You may be feeling a little lighter, a little brighter and a little clearer. Chances are your digestion is good, your sleep is restful and you are catching yourself smiling more! Remember to eat simple and clean. Our digestive system cannot digest junk. I find that many of us think we are eating clean but are actually eating foods that are wreaking havoc on our digestion and causing inflammation. Food is either fuel or inflammation. Listen to the signs and signals your body sends you.

Journal Entry: Affirmations are powerful tools to help us develop a positive attitude. An affirmation is simply a phrase or sentence that describes a clear intention. For example: I experience joy in my life or I am loved and cared for. Write an affirmation for this day.

DAY 19

Take some time for yourself and remain in silence. If you can do a day of silence, all the better. No phones, no radio and no connections. Try not to engage with others, no texting, no eye contact, no touching. Just silence. How do you feel? Maybe this is just the rest you need, or maybe there is fear in having no connection—in being silent. To turn inward and silence the senses as much as possible allows a deep rejuvenation. Try it—the rewards will be well worth it, I promise!

Journal Entry: In my silence I feel . . .

Unplug During Meals

Yes, you heard me. Put down the phone. Turn off the TV. Sit down and just enjoy the activity of eating. Give yourself some quiet time so that you can de-stress and digest.

I know life gets busy, but living and eating this way is causing you to miss the moment that you are in. If I do not give myself a little check-out time, I get tired and moody, and over time I will gain weight, feel depressed and have poor digestion.

Why? It is so simple: When the body is stressed, it cannot digest, properly function, effectively transform food into energy or perform all of its other jobs and metabolic processes.

IMPORTANT AYURVEDA PRACTICES

Take Care of Your Skin

Although we are used to thinking of nutrition as something we eat, the skin also ingests nutrients. When you slather your body with a cream or lotion, it goes directly into the bloodstream. And indeed, many medications in skin patches work this way. Today's skin care is loaded with toxins and health-disrupting chemicals that can make you sick. So, it makes sense on this cleanse to use skin care as food. Toss out the chemical toxic soup that's disguised as skin care and try these natural and synthetic-free alternatives.

Select the chemical-free face wash that is right for your dosha and start nourishing your skin immediately.

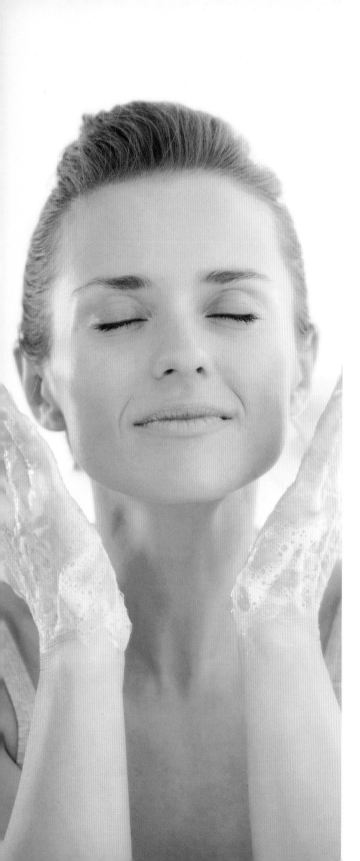

Vata Facial Wash

1 tsp almond meal
½ tsp dry milk
1 pinch raw cane sugar
Warm water, as needed

In a small bowl, mix together the almond meal, dry milk and cane sugar. Make a paste in your palm with ¼ teaspoon of the facial wash and warm water. Apply the paste all over your face and neck, gently massaging. Do not scrub. Rinse well with warm water and gently pat dry.

Pitta Facial Wash

1 tsp almond meal
½ tsp grated orange peel
½ tsp dry milk
Rosewater, as needed

In a small bowl, mix together the almond meal, orange peel and dry milk. Make a paste in your palm using ¼ teaspoon of the facial wash and rosewater. Apply the paste all over your face and neck, gently massaging. Do not scrub. Rinse well with cool water and gently pat dry.

Kapha Facial Wash

1 tsp barley meal
1 tsp grated lemon peel
½ tsp dry milk
Warm water, as needed

In a small bowl, mix together the barley meal, lemon peel and dry milk. Make a paste in your palm with ¼ teaspoon of the mixture and warm water. Apply the paste all over your face and neck, gently massaging. Do not scrub. Rinse well with warm water and gently pat dry.

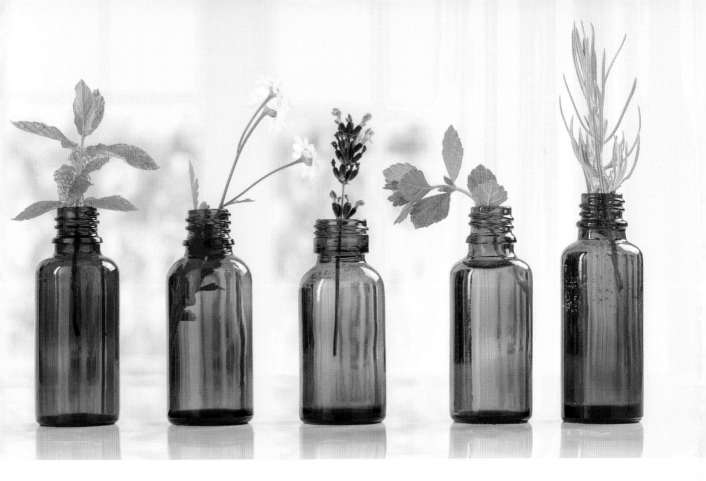

Aromatic Misters

The sense of smell is one way we can digest the world. Explore your sense of smell and observe the smells around you. Can you smell the herbs in the garden? Do you love the smell of the ocean? The cooling smells of a forest? Stop and literally smell the roses! Make an aromatic mister by adding essential oils (EO) to filtered water. These chemical-free misters are just right for your dosha and can be used anywhere.

Vata (calming and warming)

1 cup (240 ml) distilled water

3 drops neroli EO

3 drops lemon EO

2 drops jasmine EO

2 drops sandalwood EO

1 drop vanilla EO

Pitta (calming and cooling)

1 cup (240 ml) distilled water

5 drops sandalwood EO

5 drops vetiver EO

1 drop jasmine EO

Kapha (stimulating)

1 cup (240 ml) distilled water

4 drops bergamot EO

3 drops lavender EO

3 drops basil EO

Stop and Slow Down

We are all rushing: rushing to eat, to squeeze in an errand, meet a deadline or get to an appointment. So, let us slow down. Start the process with your eating.

Stop and actually sit down when you eat. Your body needs you to be calm to digest your food. If you are stressed, nervous, anxious or in fight-or-flight mode—your digestion will not work efficiently.

Before you eat, try and remember to take a deep breath. Be grateful for the food you are about to eat, and also check in with your own body. Don't shove the food into your mouth as you are running out the door or while standing at the counter as we have all done. You will be amazed by the immediate improvement you will see and feel.

Chew, Chew, Chew!

"Kerry, I am so tired and I have no energy!" I hear this from my new clients all the time. If you want more energy, then chew your food properly.

Digestion begins in your mouth. Remember when you were little and your mother would tell you to slow down and chew your food? She was right because when you do not chew your food, it sets the stage for poor digestion. And in turn, poor digestion sets the stage for digestive toxins (ama), and those let in unwanted weight gain, acne, poor sleep, hormonal issues, adrenal fatigue, constipation, IBS, low sex drive, mood swings and food allergies. Serious health issues are not far behind. Most importantly, when you do not digest properly, your body cannot transform your food into energy.

Digestion is not just about digesting the food on your plate. It is also about digesting the life you live!

ACTIVE CLEANSE MEAL PLAN

Freshly prepared foods are best, so you'll want to cook your breakfast and Kitchari (page 132) fresh each day, at whatever time works best with your schedule. While you'll want to avoid eating leftovers from previous days during this phase of the cleanse (and all throughout, if you can manage), it is acceptable to prepare all of your food for the day first thing in the morning. Garnishes such as Fresh Coriander Chutney (page 135) and Sesame Seed Chutney (page 135) can usually be refrigerated for several days without issue.

It is not uncommon to experience mild constipation during this phase of the cleanse. However, healthy elimination is critical to the detoxification process, so it is best to be proactive about relieving any discomfort as soon as you are aware of it.

Shopping List

Follow the sample meal plan that is right for your dosha and purchase the ingredients for the meals that you fancy. In addition, you will need:

- 4 lb (1.8 kg) basmati rice
- 2 lb (910 g) mung beans
- Vegetables for Kitchari (page 132)—see the right vegetables for your dosha
- Spice mix for your dosha (page 32)
- 1 bag rolled oats

ACTIVE CLEANSE RECIPES

Each of the following recipes were designed specifically for the active cleanse portion of your 25-day cleanse. As in Phase 1, the recipes are written for Vata with adaptations given for Pitta and Kapha.

Meal Plan for Active-Cleanse

	DAY 12	DAY 13	DAY 14	DAY 15
Breakfast	Dosha Tea (page 31) Baked Apples with Dates, Cinnamon and Cardamom (page 127)	Dosha Tea (page 31) Spiced Amaranth Porridge (page 128)	Dosha Tea (page 31) Not Your Mother's Oatmeal (page 43)	Dosha Tea (page 31) Breakfast Rice (page 52)
Mid-Morning	Dosha Tea (page 31)			
Lunch	Kitchari (page 132)			
Mid-Afternoon	Dosha Tea (page 31)			
Supper	Kitchari (page 132)			

	DAY 16	DAY 17	DAY 18
Breakfast	Dosha Tea (page 31) Baked Coconut-Apple Oatmeal (page 131)	Dosha Tea (page 31) Chia Breakfast Bowl (page 124)	Dosha Tea (page 31) Detox Breakfast Stew (page 61)
Mid-Morning	Dosha Tea (page 31)		
Lunch	Kitchari (page 132)		
Mid-Afternoon	Dosha Tea (page 31)		
Supper	Kitchari (page 132)		

CHIA BREAKFAST BOWL

Chia seeds are cooling and have the ability to retain water in our bodies. This keeps us hydrated at all tissue levels, especially during the summer months. Chia seeds help us beat the heat, maintain agility and fight off fatigue. Chia seeds are also one of the best foods with omega-3 fatty acid, which increases immunity, balances blood pressure and keeps the heart healthy and fit. Finally, chia seeds are rich in fiber, which helps stimulate a healthy digestive system and prevents any gastrointestinal disorders. Chia seeds reduce Vata, are cooling for Pitta and help with Kapha.

YIELD: 1 serving

¾ cup (180 ml) filtered water

½ tsp vanilla extract

1 tsp maple syrup

1½ tsp chia seeds

¼ tsp ground cinnamon

¼ tsp ground cardamom

¼ tsp ground nutmeg

Place the water, vanilla, syrup, chia, cinnamon, cardamom and nutmeg in a bowl and stir to combine them. Cover and refrigerate it overnight to let the chia seeds absorb the liquid.

Dosha Adaptations

RECIPE WRITTEN FOR VATA.
PITTA: Omit the nutmeg.
KAPHA: Substitute raw honey for the maple syrup.

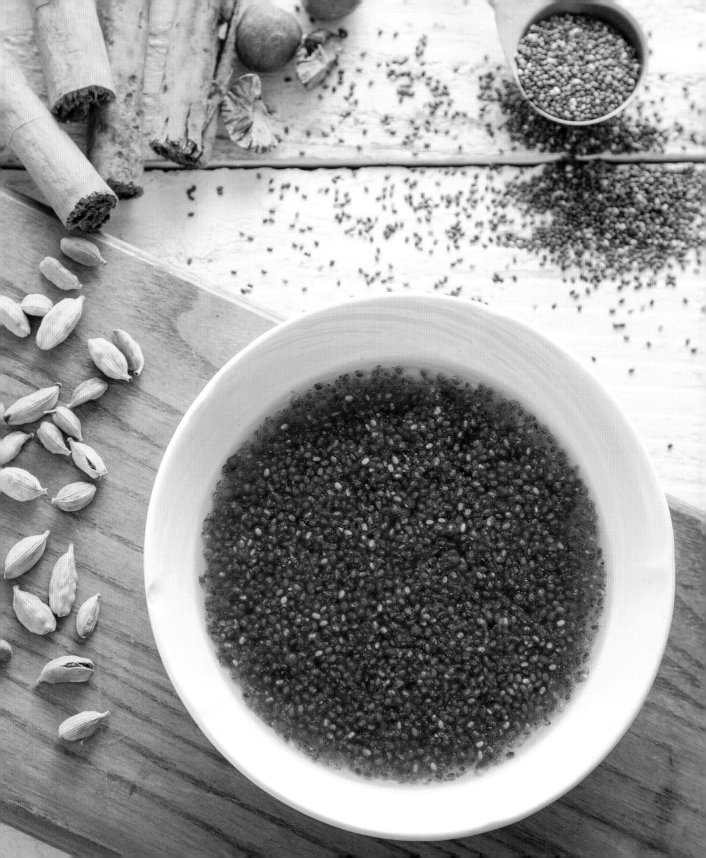

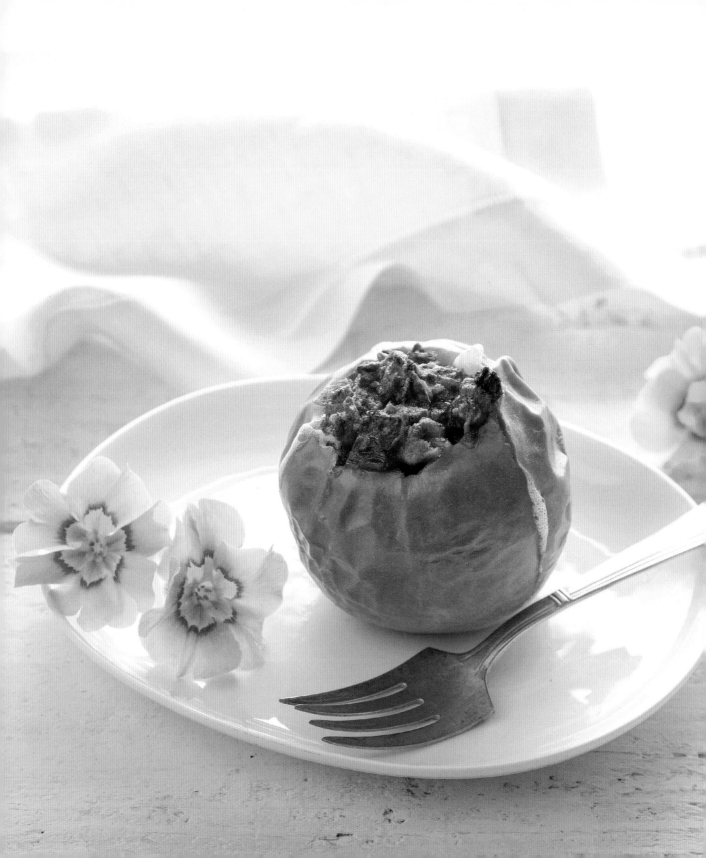

BAKED APPLES WITH DATES, CINNAMON AND CARDAMOM

This comforting and warming dish is great for balancing Vatas. Cooked fruit is so much easier to digest than raw fruit, and combined with the warming spices, it helps improve digestion.

YIELD: 1 serving

1 green apple, cored
½ tsp ground cinnamon
¼ tsp ground cardamom
¼ tsp freshly grated ginger
2 dates, pitted and chopped
Honey, as desired

Preheat the oven to 350°F (180°C).

Place the apple in a small baking dish and add a little water. Combine the cinnamon, cardamom, ginger, dates and honey in a bowl and then spoon it into the center of the apple. Bake for 35 to 40 minutes, or until cooked through. Eat warm.

Dosha Adaptations

RECIPE WRITTEN FOR VATA.
PITTA: Omit the ginger.
KAPHA: Substitute raisins for the dates.

SPICED AMARANTH PORRIDGE

You may not have come across amaranth before, but it is an easily digestible grain that is packed with protein. Amaranth is gluten-free and a great alternative to oatmeal. This grain can stimulate growth and repair, reduce inflammation, boost bone strength and help lower blood pressure. The warming digestive spices will make your tummy glow so you'll feel happy until lunchtime.

YIELD: 2 servings

1 tbsp (15 g) ghee

¼ tsp ground ginger

¼ tsp ground cinnamon

¼ tsp ground cardamom

Pinch of nutmeg

Pinch of cloves

Pinch of allspice

1 star anise

1½ cups (360 ml) water

¾ cup (135 g) amaranth

Pinch of salt

½ tsp vanilla extract

Handful of dried raisins or dates

Almond milk, for serving

Dried persimmons, for garnishing (optional)

In a saucepan, heat the ghee, and then add the ginger, cinnamon, cardamom, nutmeg, cloves, allspice and star anise. Stir for 2 minutes, or until fragrant. Add the water, amaranth, salt and vanilla and bring it to a boil, stirring. Add the raisins. Reduce the heat and simmer, covered, for 20 minutes, or until it's smooth and creamy.

Remove the star anise and serve with almond milk. Sprinkle with dried persimmons, if desired.

Dosha Adaptations

RECIPE WRITTEN FOR VATA.
PITTA: Omit the cloves and use coconut milk instead of the almond milk.
KAPHA: Use cranberries instead of raisins or dates. Use soy milk instead of almond milk.

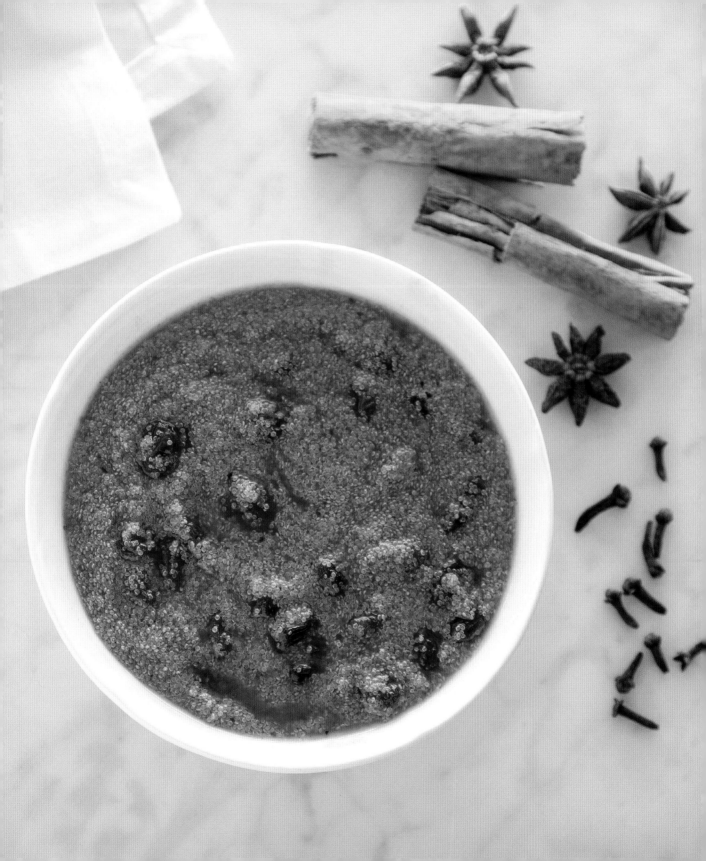

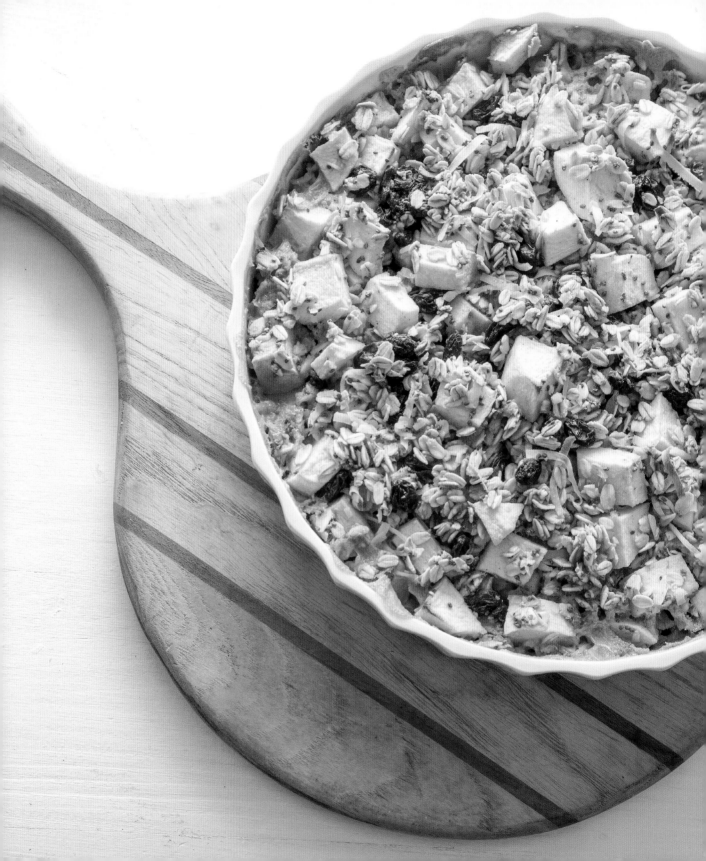

BAKED COCONUT-APPLE OATMEAL

This is the perfect breakfast for a chilly morning. It is packed full of fiber and flavor. The oats provide a grounding base and the warming digestive spices mean your digestion will be happy all morning!

YIELD: 4 servings

2 tbsp (20 g) chia seeds

¼ cup (60 ml) water

2 cups (200 g) rolled oats

2 large green apples, diced

2 tbsp (10 g) unsweetened coconut flakes

½ cup (70 g) raisins

1 tsp baking powder

1 tbsp (9 g) ground cinnamon

½ tsp ground cardamom

¼ tsp sea salt

2 cups (480 ml) almond milk

2 tbsp (40 g) maple syrup

2 tsp (10 ml) vanilla extract

Preheat the oven to 350°F (180°C). Lightly oil a medium baking pan.

In a bowl, combine the chia seeds and water. Set it aside for 5 minutes.

In a large bowl, combine the oats, apples, coconut flakes, raisins, baking powder, cinnamon, cardamom and salt.

In a small bowl, whisk together the almond milk, maple syrup, vanilla and the chia mixture. Fold the wet ingredients into the oat mixture and transfer it to the baking dish. Bake for 45 minutes, or until golden brown on top. Remove the dish from the oven and allow it to cool for 10 minutes before serving.

Dosha Adaptations

RECIPE WRITTEN FOR VATA.

PITTA: Substitute coconut milk for the almond milk.

KAPHA: Use cranberries instead of raisins. Use millet instead of oats. Use soy milk instead of almond milk. Use a few drops of liquid stevia instead of maple syrup.

KITCHARI

Kitchari is a potent blood purifier and also supports proper kidney function. Made with basmati rice and mung beans, it is a great source of protein that detoxifies and reduces free radicals. It also nourishes and rejuvenates the digestive system. Known as a heavy metal stripper and pesticide chelator, kitchari is especially helpful for the reproductive organs, liver and the thyroid. The digestive spices work on igniting your agni and burning off ama. That will, in turn, have you feeling peaceful, calm, clear and focused.

YIELD: 4 servings

1 cup (185 g) uncooked white basmati rice, rinsed

1 cup (200 g) split mung beans, rinsed

4 cups (960 ml) filtered water

1 zucchini, chopped

1 small sweet potato, peeled and chopped

2 cups (250 g) cleansing veggies (your choice, see notes)

2 tbsp (30 g) ghee, plus more for garnish

2 tbsp (20 g) pumpkin seeds

2 tbsp (6 g) chopped scallions

2 tsp (6 g) dosha-specific spice mix (page 32)

½ cup (120 ml) coconut milk

2 tbsp (30 ml) lemon juice

½ tsp maple syrup

Salt and pepper, as desired

Fresh cilantro, for garnishing

Fresh Coriander Chutney or Sesame Seed Chutney, as desired (page 135)

In a large saucepan, add the rice, mung beans and water and bring it to a boil over high heat. Reduce the heat to low and simmer, covered, for 10 minutes. Add even layers of zucchini, sweet potato and cleansing veggies on top of the rice mixture. Cover the pan and cook until the rice mixture has absorbed all the water, about 20 minutes.

In a skillet, heat the ghee over medium heat. Add the pumpkin seeds and scallions and cook, stirring, for 4 minutes, or until the seeds turn light brown. Stir in the dosha spice mix, coconut milk, lemon juice and maple syrup and cook for 20 to 25 minutes.

Pour the scallion mixture over the rice and stir to blend them well. Season to taste with salt and pepper. Garnish with cilantro and ghee and serve with your choice of chutney (page 135), if desired.

Dosha Adaptations

This is truly a tridoshic meal that is good for all doshas.

NOTES: Try to remember this if you get tired of eating the Kitchari twice a day: It is really the mind that is rebelling, not your digestive system. Add some variety by creating tasty side dishes such as steamed vegetables.

Cleansing vegetables include cauliflower, cabbage, broccoli, Brussels sprouts, carrots, artichokes, asparagus, celery, bok choy, green beans, okra, scallions, kale, fennel and watercress. Also, you can top your Kitchari with one of the chutneys (page 135) for some variety.

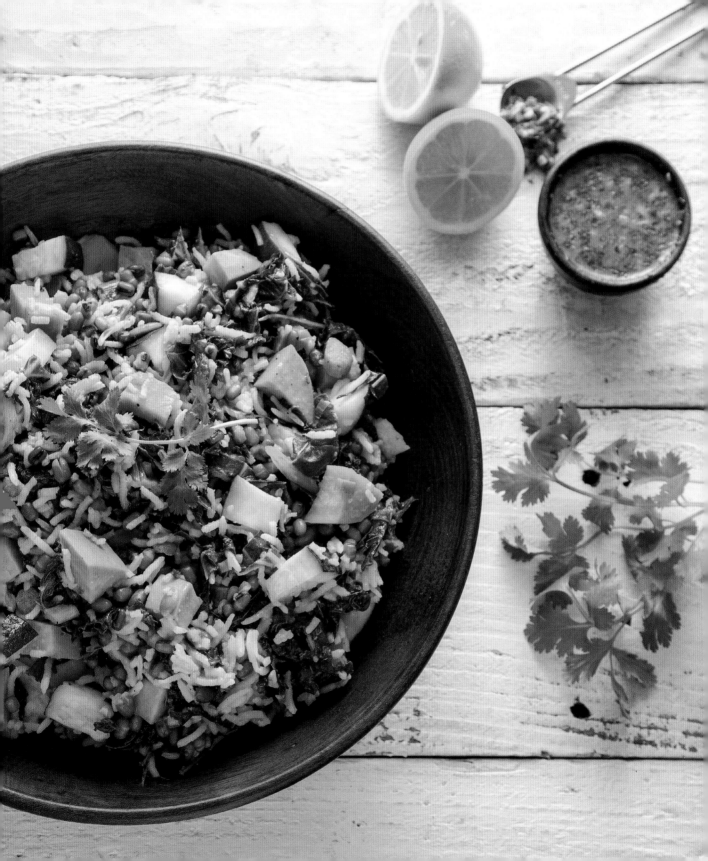

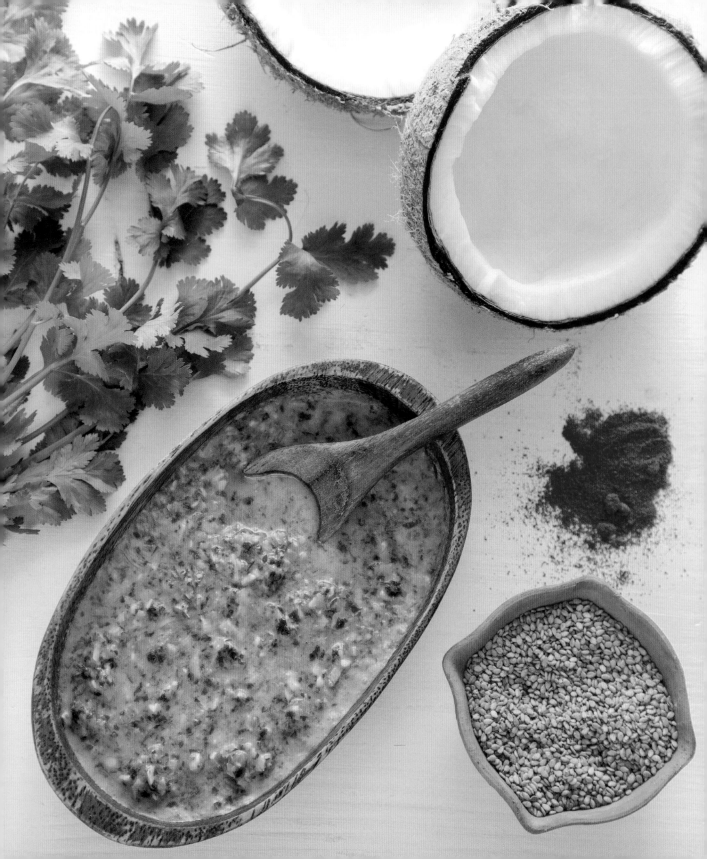

SPICE IT UP WITH CHUTNEY

Sometimes it is nice to have variety, so if you want to spice up your kitchari, you can add one of the following chutneys. Chutneys are traditionally part of an Ayurvedic meal because they not only add delicious taste, but they also add nutrition and improve digestion by stimulating agni (digestive fire). Just add a teaspoon or two to spice up your next meal. The Fresh Coriander Chutney is especially useful for reducing excess Pitta, while the Sesame Seed Chutney is good for people with Vata and Kapha imbalance.

FRESH CORIANDER CHUTNEY

YIELD: 1 cup (140 g)

¼ cup (60 ml) fresh lemon juice

¼ cup (60 ml) water

1 bunch fresh coriander leaves and stems

⅓ cup (25 g) grated coconut

2 tbsp (18 g) chopped fresh ginger

1 tsp raw honey

1 tsp natural mineral salt

In a blender, process the lemon juice, water and coriander until the coriander is chopped. Add the coconut, ginger, honey and salt and process until it is like a paste. This chutney can be stored in a covered container in the refrigerator for up to 1 week. For a silkier texture, use only the leaves of the fresh coriander stalks.

Dosha Adaptations

RECIPE WRITTEN FOR VATA.
PITTA: Recommended for Pittas.
KAPHA AND VATA: Kaphas and Vatas would do better with the Sesame Seed Chutney.

SESAME SEED CHUTNEY

YIELD: 1 cup (140 g)

1 cup (140 g) roasted and ground sesame seeds

1 tsp cayenne pepper

¼ tsp natural mineral salt

In a blender, process the sesame seeds, cayenne pepper and salt until combined. This chutney can be stored in a covered container in the refrigerator for up to 1 week.

Dosha Adaptations

RECIPE WRITTEN FOR VATA.
PITTA: Pittas would do better with the Fresh Coriander Chutney.
KAPHA: This is a great chutney for Kaphas.

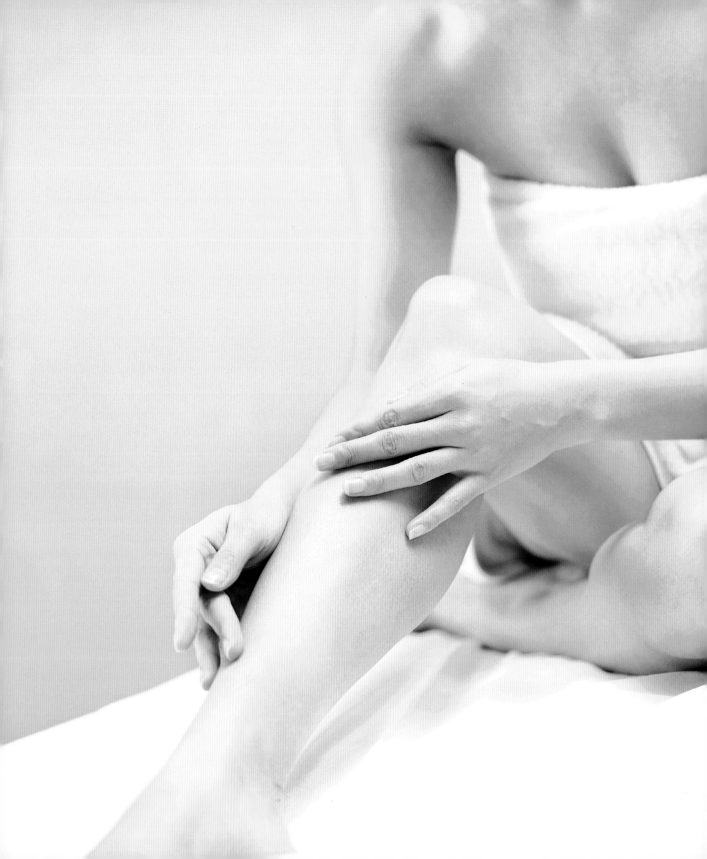

SELF-CARE

During this phase of the cleanse, self-care practices such as abhyanga (ayurvedic self-massage with oil), yoga postures, pranayama (breathwork) and taking supportive herbs can enhance the impact of the cleanse. These practices will also help rid yourself of toxic ways of thinking about your body and get you in the habit of loving your body, which is the ultimate commitment to yourself, your life and your health.

Right now, take a deep breath, uncross anything you have crossed (arms, legs, hands) and close your eyes. As you exhale, take a mental look at you: not your bad hair day, or the lines around your eyes or the latest inch you can pinch. Take a look at *you* and see how strong you are, the people you have hugged with your arms, the walks you have done with your legs . . . Go deeper now and observe all your organs working in union to make *you*. Love yourself because you are perfect just as you are now!

Abhyanga Oil Self-Massage

Yes, you are going to get oily. Don't worry, you and your skin will love it. Abhyanga benefits all three doshas, but you will need to use the right oil for your dosha. It's a head-to-toe massage and the benefits are that oiling nourishes the skin but most importantly calms the nervous system, helps remove toxins from the blood stream and is incredibly nourishing for the tissues.

Vatas benefit the most from oiling as it's calming and grounding. Use sesame oil or almond oil and light strokes. Pittas need a lighter oil, such as coconut or almond oil. You will benefit from adding more pressure to your strokes.

Vatas and Pittas benefit greatly from abhyanga, but Kaphas will need to dry-brush instead. Using cotton gloves on your hands, start with your feet and work toward the heart, brushing with a firm and steady pressure. In general, use circular strokes over the joints and tummy and long, vertical strokes over the limbs.

After you choose the oil that is right for your dosha, warm it by placing the oil in a plastic bottle and adding the bottle to a bowl of very hot water. Apply the oil starting from the toes, using steady pressure. Use long strokes toward the heart on your legs and thighs. Use a circular motion for the joints like knees and ankles. Use a circular motion on your belly and long strokes as you move up your body.

From your hands, massage them gently and use long strokes on the arms toward the heart. Try and reach every part of your body. You can use the oil on your face and neck and even hair and scalp. This type of oiling helps with hair growth and thickness too.

This is time for self-care. Love your body as you oil it. It has served you well. This is an opportunity to really nurture all your parts—even those that you normally try to ignore. This is all part of healing.

Once covered, take a hot shower and allow the water to wash off some of the oil. I recommend avoiding soap, as the detergent will just remove the oil. However, if you need to use soap on certain areas, go ahead! After your shower, gently pat dry. Again, you don't want to remove the oil with the towel. Love how soft your skin feels, how your muscles are less tense and your mind is calmer.

Cleansing Yoga Sequence

This sequence is designed to relax, cool and calm your energy. Using slow and steady movements, this noncompetitive approach will focus you on just being present—on *being* and not *doing*. The twists in the practice will aid detoxification of the liver and blood but will still keep you cool. This yoga practice is a bit longer than in the other phases (40 to 45 minutes) and will have you balanced rather than pushing. Simply move from pose to pose and don't worry if it takes time to figure out how to move from pose to pose. This isn't a race! If you would like to join me with your yoga or meditation, go to www.theholistichighway.com/bookspecial and type in the password "Ayurveda." Here you'll find videos and audio to accompany the book, and we can do this together.

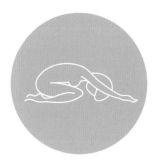

Child Pose (2 minutes)

1. Press your bottom back to sit on your heels and lay your chest on your legs, resting your forehead on the ground. If your bottom does not quite reach your heels, just place a folded blanket on your thighs, so you can enjoy the pose.

2. Put your arms and hands on the floor with your palms facing up with elbows slightly bent. Breathe deeply into the belly about 10 times.

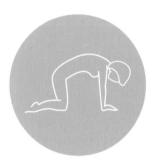

Cat Stretch (1 minute)

1. Come up onto your hands and knees. Place your shoulders directly above your wrists and your hips directly over your knees. Spread your fingers open like a fan and press the entire surface of your hands into the floor.

2. Inhale, drawing your tailbone toward the sky and dipping your abdomen toward the earth. Continue this movement until your chest and gaze are moving upwards.

3. Exhale, drawing your tailbone back toward the ground as you lift your navel up toward the ceiling. Bring your chin toward your chest to lengthen the back of your neck. Repeat 5 times.

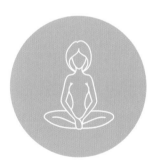

Happy Hip Opener (1 minute)

1. Come up onto your knees and then swing your legs out in front. Sit on the floor with your knees bent and out to the sides, soles of your feet together. You may find it easier to sit on a folded blanket or cushion.

2. Inhale and lengthen your spine, exhale—and hinge forward from the hips. Allow your chest to reach for the floor and just relax here for 4 to 5 breaths.

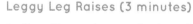

Leggy Leg Raises (3 minutes)

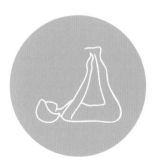

1. Transition onto your back and straighten your legs. Inhale—bend the right knee and take hold of the right foot with the right hand. If needed, use a belt or strap around the foot.

2. As you exhale, straighten the right knee, pushing the right heel up toward the ceiling. Make sure your hips stay on the mat and your left leg stays on the floor. The right arm remains straight. Breathe gently and smoothly for 5 breaths.

3. On an exhalation, bring the right leg back by bending the knee first and then straighten. Simply note how this leg has lengthened.

4. Repeat on the other side. Repeat the whole pose several times.

Head to Knee (2 minutes)

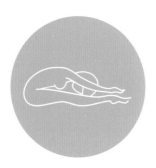

1. From a seated position, inhale and bend the left knee, pulling the left foot toward your upper right thigh. Face the right leg. Exhale—lengthen the right leg and relax your body over the extended leg. Keeping your spine long, enjoy the deep stretch and stay here for 5 breaths.

2. On an inhale, come back up to center. Bring the two legs back together, take 2 deep breaths and repeat on the other side.

Twstin' and Rockin' (2 minutes)

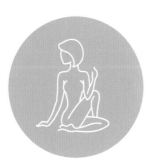

1. In a seated position with legs straight out in front of you, bend the left leg and place the foot on the outside of your right leg. Press your fingertips on the floor and elongate the spine. Hug the outside of your left leg with your right arm. Exhale—twisting your torso to the left beginning the twist from the base of the spine.

2. With each exhalation, lift the spine and ribs as you continue to twist. The twist naturally massages all your internal organs. Gently twist the neck to look over your left shoulder, hold for 5 breaths, breathing deeply into the belly.

3. On an exhalation, gently release the twist, starting with the neck and ending with the base of your spine. Take a breath and repeat on the other side.

Back Vinyasa (2 minutes)

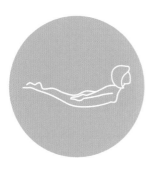

1. Lie facedown on the floor with your legs together and the tops of your feet on the floor. Tighten the backs of your legs. Stretch your arms back along the floor.

2. On your next inhalation, lift your legs, chest, arms and head off the floor. Make sure you look just ahead of you on the floor (no neck strains needed). Take 3 breaths here and slowly lower down. Windshield-wiper the legs side to side. Repeat 4 times.

Child Pose (2 minutes)

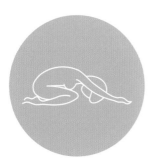

1. Press your bottom back to sit on your heels and lay your chest on your legs, resting your forehead on the ground. If your bottom does not quite reach your heels, just place a folded blanket on your thighs, so you can enjoy the pose.

2. Put your arms and hands on the floor with your palms facing up with elbows slightly bent. Breathe deeply into the belly about 10 times.

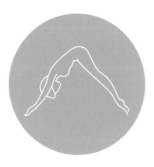

Downward Facing Dog (1 minute)

1. From Child Pose, come into the tabletop position, on your hands and knees with a flat back. As you exhale—come onto the balls of your feet and straighten your legs. Keep your heels up as you lengthen the spine, the arms, shoulders and torso.

2. Bring your sitting bones up to the ceiling, making a straight line from hands to tailbone.

3. Holding the straight line, slowly lower your heels to the floor, but only if that works for you. Hold the pose for 4 breaths.

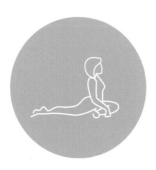

Totally Pigeon (3 minutes)

1. In Downward Facing Dog, inhale, bend the right knee forward and place it between your hands.

2. Bring your pelvis forward, keeping the hips even. Exhale and stretch the left thigh back, placing the left knee and left thigh on the floor.

3. Inhale—lengthen your spine, exhale and allow your torso to elongate and gently fold over toward your mat. You may prop your forehead on your hands or on a block if your forehead is not reaching the floor. Stay here for 10 breaths and breathe into the stretch. On the exhale relax further into the pose.

4. On the inhalation, come out of the pose by placing your hands on the ground, straighten the back leg and lift your bent leg and transition back into Downward Facing Dog. Repeat on the other side.

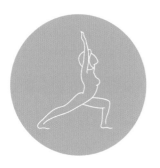

Stretch It Again (1 minute)

1. Inhale as you step your left leg and foot forward 5 to 6 feet (1.5 to 1.8 m). Bend your left leg at a 90-degree angle. Your right leg should be straight.

2. Open your chest forward and relax your hips down to the floor. Stay here for 4 breaths.

3. Exhale as you step your left leg back to Downward Facing Dog and take 2 breaths here.

4. Inhale, step your right leg and foot forward and repeat the pose. End up in Downward Facing Dog.

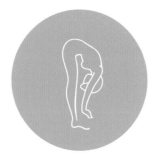

Just Hangin' (1 minute)

1. Spread your feet to each side of the mat and slowly walk your hands to your feet. Allow your torso to hang forward toward the floor. Inhale—maintaining the forward fold. Exhale—and relax your hanging torso even more. Release and relax your neck and shoulders. Stay here for 10 breaths.

2. Slowly with your knees bent, tuck your tailbone under as you slowly unroll your spine to a standing position. Take at least 45 seconds to do this.

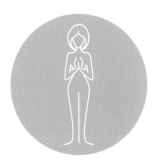

Strong as a Mountain (1 minute)

1. Stand up with your feet parallel and your knees together. Interlace your fingers together so your palms are facing the ceiling.

2. On an inhalation, rise up to the balls of your feet and lift your palms up to the ceiling. Hold for a minute before exhaling and lowering your heels to the floor. Repeat 8 more times.

Twist That Triangle (2 minutes)

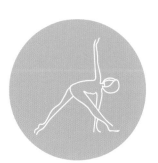

1. From Strong as a Mountain pose, spread your legs 3 to 4 feet (0.9 to 1.2 m) apart on an exhalation. Turn your legs, feet and torso to the right so your hips face the right. Inhale—allow your arms to come up to shoulder level, extending horizontally from your shoulder to your fingertips.

2. Exhale—turn your left hip, abdomen and torso toward your right thigh. Press your left heel into the floor and twist so that your chest is turned toward your right leg. Inhale as you bring your left hand down to the floor on the outside of your right foot. With each exhalation twist just a little farther. Stay here for 4 breaths.

3. On your next inhalation, with your left arm extended, bring your torso up to standing. As you exhale, turn your feet forward and jump or step back to Strong as a Mountain pose. Take a couple of breaths here.

Tree Balance (1 minute)

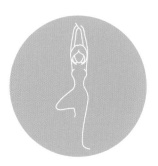

1. Stand with your weight equally distributed between both feet. Begin to shift your body weight toward the right foot. Place the ball of your left foot to the right ankle or on the side of the right calf or inner thigh (not beside the right knee). Keep your pelvis square to the front of the room.

2. Bring your hands together in front of your heart or above your head. Breathe comfortably as you balance on one leg. Smile and stay as long as you can. Repeat on the other side.

Triangle (2 minutes)

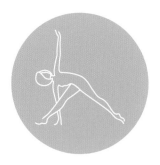

1. Stand with both feet together. Move the left leg approximately 3 to 4 feet (0.9 to 1.2 m) to the side and place the left foot on a forward angle of about 45 degrees.

2. Inhale—raise both arms up to shoulder height. Exhale—shift the weight of your pelvis toward the left as you reach to the side with the torso and right arm (keeping both sides of the torso long and even).

3. Place the right hand on the right leg without collapsing your body weight into it. Look up toward the left hand. Breathe here for 5 full breaths.

4. Inhale—to press into your feet, engage your core and return upright. Exhale—lower your hands to your hips. Inhale—step the left foot forward beside the right foot. Repeat on the second side.

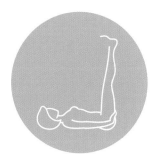

Wind Down Waterfall (3–5 minutes)

1. Sit sideways with your right hip against the wall.

2. Use the support of your hands to gently roll yourself onto your back with your legs up against the wall. Your sitting bones should touch the wall. Relax your entire body as your legs stay extended up the wall in alignment with your hips. Your arms are comfortably out to the side, palms up.

3. To come out of this restorative pose, bend your knees and push your feet against the wall to slide the body away from the wall. Then turn to your right side and rest here for a few minutes. Use your arms to push yourself up to sitting.

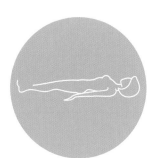

Save-It Savasana (10 minutes)

1. Lie down comfortably on your back with your legs extended. Cover yourself with a blanket if you are apt to get cold.

2. Pull the shoulders down and back as you lengthen your arms along your side, palms up. Lengthen your neck. Inhale deeply, exhale and allow your whole body to relax.

3. Systematically relax each part of your body beginning with your feet. Relax your toes, then ankles, then calves, knees and hips, all while moving your awareness up through your body, consciously relaxing any stress or tight spots along the way. Keep your breath deep and natural and allow yourself to surrender into the stillness of this pose.

4. After about 10 minutes, slowly deepen your breath, wiggle your fingers and toes, bring some movement back into your body by stretching in any way that feels good to you.

5. Roll onto your right side, stay there for a couple of minutes and then use your hands to push yourself into an upright seated position.

White Light Meditation

If you would like to join me with your yoga or meditation, go to www.theholistichighway.com/bookspecial and type in the password "Ayurveda." Here you'll find videos and audio to accompany the book, and we can do this together.

Your light is seen, your heart is known, your soul is cherished by more people than you might imagine. You would be astonished if you knew how many others have been touched in wonderful ways by you. If you knew how many people feel so much for you, you would be shocked. You are far more wonderful than you think you are. Rest with that. Rest easy with that. Breathe again. You are doing fine. More than fine. Better than fine. You're doing great. So relax and love yourself today.

Pranayama: Kapalabhati Breathing

Kapawhat?! Kapal-a-bah-tee.

Kapalabhati is a breathing exercise that is literally translated as "glowing" or "shining" skull. It's the best because it purifies the mind by forcefully expelling all toxins. The breathing itself is a series of forceful exhalations one after the other while never intentionally inhaling. The body will automatically inhale for us—we don't need to worry about it.

Benefits of kapalabhati:

* It's weight reducing! Who knew that just by breathing you could lose weight?

* It improves your respiratory system.

* It stimulates your digestive system. Remember, we are what we digest, so we need to digest food properly. This will help!

* It stimulates the circulatory system.

* It improves mood—calms anxiety and reduces depression. Who wouldn't want to do this?

* It helps bring higher awareness as it focuses our mind on pure and right intention.

Here's how to do it:

1. Sit with legs crossed in a lotus-like position, or if sitting in a chair, place both feet on the ground.

2. Keep your spine straight and chest open, as if a string is going from your butt up through the top of your head and holding you straight.

3. With hands on your diaphragm, inhale while ballooning the belly.

4. Start! Forcefully exhale, using the diaphragm and count, 1–2–3–4–5. (You will automatically inhale, but focus on the exhale.)

5. Take a rest when you are tired and repeat the cycle 3 times. Even with just 2 minutes of this a day, you will notice the benefits.

NOTE: Do this daily in the morning if you can, before breakfast. Wait 2 hours if after a meal so you won't cramp up. Trust me. And when first beginning this practice, start with a count of 20 to 30, and then rest. See how you feel. This is very individual depending on your cardiovascular condition, so take it easy if you haven't done exercise in a while. Or if that was a piece of cake, try doing this for 45 seconds or 1 minute.

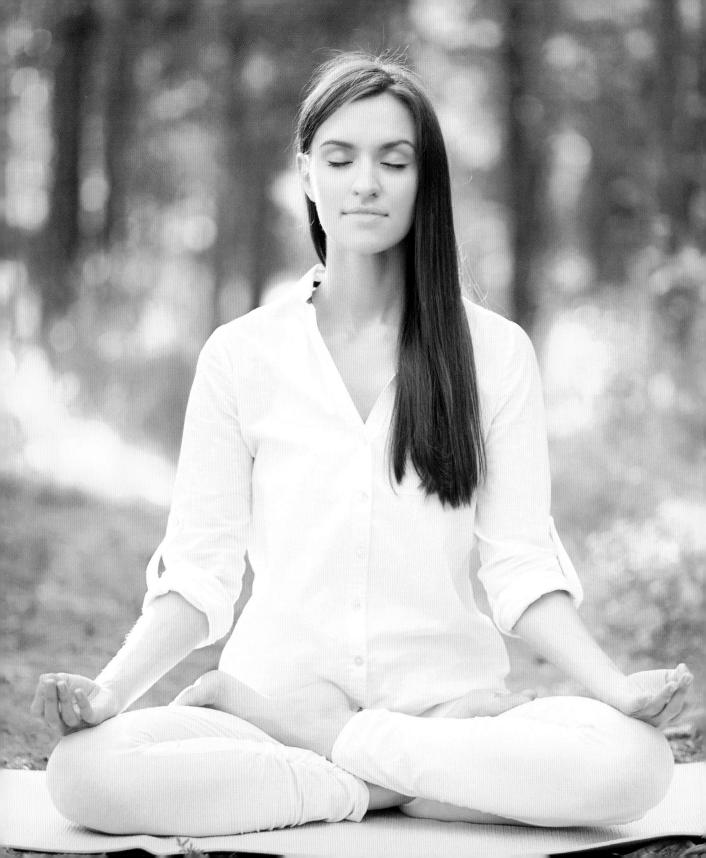

Chapter 4

PHASE 3
DAYS 20 TO 25

"Take your place in the world. Know you are part of a complete universe.
But remember, you are a complete universe, too." —Melody Beattie

POST-CLEANSE AND REINTRODUCTION

I really want to stress to you that coming out of the cleanse is just as important as the cleanse itself. As you finish the cleanse, don't immediately jump back into your normal routine. This will shock your system and can undo the benefits of your cleanse. The trick is to ease back into a healthy diet and your normal activities.

For many, this is actually the most challenging phase of the entire cleanse. It can feel like we've come through the hard part, and after days of Kitchari (page 132), we are often craving some substance and stimulation in our diets. Therefore, it is extremely important to mentally prepare for this phase. Think of it as an essential part of—rather than a gradual transition out of—the cleanse.

You may also find it helpful to plan a menu for this phase in advance. Choose meals that you will find delicious and exciting so that you are not tempted to dive right into overly complex and difficult-to-digest foods. This is not the time to celebrate with pizza and a beer! Remember, the longer your cleanse, the more time your body will need to diversify your diet and strengthen agni. Go slowly and your agni will emerge from the cleanse much stronger, which means much better health moving forward.

DAILY ROUTINE

As you follow your daily routine, take a look at the day-by-day suggestions for your post-cleanse during days 20 to 25.

At this time, you will:

- Reintroduce a variety of grains (quinoa, barley, brown rice) and healthy proteins like nuts, legumes and eggs.

- Eat your fruit separately from other foods and vegetables.

- Check in and see how you are feeling. To help you in this part of the cleanse, it is very useful to keep a food journal (page 210). This way, you can see if any particular food is causing stress in the body.

- Continue taking triphala for up to 3 months afterwards if you suffer from any gas, bloating or constipation.

- Continue with foods and activities that replenish your body. This can include the daily routines you have developed as well as the warm sesame oil or coconut oil massage.

Phase 3 Daily Routine

	VATA	PITTA	KAPHA
Wake Up	½ hour before sunrise (in spring and summer in the Northern Hemisphere, feel free to get up just before sunrise)	1 hour before sunrise (in spring and summer in the Northern Hemisphere, feel free to get up ½ hour before sunrise)	1½ hours before sunrise (in spring and summer in the Northern Hemisphere, feel free to get up 45 minutes before sunrise)
Drink	Warm water with lemon juice and ginger and maple syrup as a sweetener or Vata Cleansing Tea (page 31)	Room temperature water with lime juice and maple syrup as a sweetener or Pitta Cooling Tea (page 31)	Warm water with lemon juice, ginger tea and honey or Kapha Stimulating Tea (page 31)
Nose	Add a few drops of sesame oil or nasya oil into both nostrils (see page 35).		
Exercise	Follow Yoga Sequence (page 170).		
Shower	Massage with sesame oil before taking a hot shower or bath.	Massage with coconut oil before taking a warm/cool shower or bath.	Massage with mustard oil before taking a hot shower or bath.
Facial Serum	Vata Facial Serum (page 33)	Pitta Facial Serum (page 33)	Kapha Facial Serum (page 33)
Meditation Practice	Spend 15 minutes minimum on your daily spiritual practice. See journal suggestions.		
Breakfast	Follow a balancing breakfast for your dosha.		
Mid-Morning	Vata Cleansing Tea (page 31)	Pitta Cooling Tea (page 31)	Kapha Stimulating Tea (page 31)
Lunch (12 p.m. to 2 p.m.)	Kitchari (page 132) with Vata Spice (page 32) Take a few minutes to rest after lunch.	Kitchari (page 132) with Pitta Spice (page 32) Take a few minutes to walk after your meal.	Take 2 trikatu tablets. Kitchari (page 132) with Kapha Spice (page 32) Take a brisk walk after your meal.

	VATA	**PITTA**	**KAPHA**
Mid-Afternoon	Ojas-Building Snack (pages 158–65) and Vata Cleansing Tea (page 31)	Ojas-Building Snack (pages 158–65) and Pitta Cooling Tea (page 31)	Kapha Stimulating Tea (page 31)
Dinner (5:30 p.m. to 7:30 p.m.)	Follow a balancing meal for your dosha. Take a few minutes to rest after dinner.	Follow a balancing meal for your dosha. Take a few minutes to walk after your meal.	Follow a balancing meal for your dosha. Take a brisk walk after your meal.
Sunset	Gentle stretching or take a rejuvenating walk.	Take a walk.	Take a brisk walk.
Journal Practice	See journal suggestions.		
Nighttime	Take 2 triphala tablets or 1 tsp triphala powder in warm water.	Take 2 triphala tablets or 1 tsp triphala powder in warm water.	Take 2 triphala tablets or 1 tsp triphala powder in warm water.
Massage	Massage soles of feet with sesame oil.	Massage soles of feet with coconut oil.	Massage soles of feet with mustard oil.
Essential Oil	Add 1 drop of lavender to pillow for restful sleep.	Add 1 drop of sandalwood for cooling and revitalizing sleep.	Add 1 drop of bergamot for sleep.
Mantra Before Sleep	Let go of worries and conflicts of the day.	Let go of what I can't control.	Let go of what does not serve me anymore.

DAY 20

Start your day with your morning warm water with lemon and a slice of ginger. This will keep stimulating your digestive fire. Add a morning breakfast that is right for your dosha. Don't forget to take your Ojas-Building Snack (pages 158–65) with you to work. What can you let go of that no longer nourishes you? Perhaps there is some "stuff" or friendship or relationship, or even a job that is holding you down and not allowing you to feel truly nourished anymore. When you move out the stuff that you no longer need, the vacuum created can be filled with healthy relationships that support and honor you. You deserve that.

Journal Entry: What will you open yourself up to once you have cleared the space?

DAY 21

How are you feeling today? Still scraping your tongue? Still oiling? Don't be in too much of a rush to add caffeine back to your diet. Ask yourself if this is a habit you can do without. Eat your Kitchari (page 132) for one meal a day. Are you enjoying adding back some variety in your foods?

Journal Entry: How do you like to best express yourself? How are you showing up in the world? You have the power to be the best version of yourself. Who is that person?

DAY 22

Allow yourself enough time to do your morning and evening practices. Are they becoming more habitual now? It takes at least 30 days for something to become a habit. Stay the course and all these wonderful things you have implemented will become more ingrained into your daily life.

Journal Entry: The habits I want to stick with are . . . I am most challenged by . . . Are there ways you can overcome these challenges?

DAY 23

Are you using your health tracker (page 209)? Are there any patterns you are noticing over the days? Pay attention to any signs of poor digestion, gas and bloating, heartburn, diarrhea and constipation or burping. Use your health tracker to determine which foods may be causing problems and add them back into your diet more slowly. You might want to wait a week or so to add them back in.

Journal Entry: How are you incorporating your self-care? What is it you do to honor and love yourself?

DAY 24

Make sure you are eating all meals away from the TV, computer or phone. As you eat today, pay special attention to the smells, colors and presentation of your food. Eat slowly and absorb these sights and smells. Give thanks for this food that is nourishing you through all the five senses.

Journal Entry: Write down your daily practices, including your morning and evening rituals. How have these changed you?

DAY 25

Wow, you did it! It is the last day of the cleanse. You have reset and restored your digestion. Remember that picture you took at the beginning of the cleanse? Take another and compare it. How have you changed? Enjoy your last day of Kitchari (page 132) and know that you can always come back to this comfort food for a few days anytime you want to reset your digestion. Begin to add more variety to your meals by following the sample meal plan for your dosha. Continue taking the triphala for another month if there are any signs of digestive problems like indigestion, gas, bloating or constipation. Give yourself a big hug—there is no better care than self-care and you thought enough of yourself to give it the first step to great health. Congratulations!

Journal Entry: How do you feel now you have committed to working on you for 25 days? Write down all the ways this cleanse has changed you both physically and emotionally. What will you take forward with you?

Post-Digestive Effect

Vipaka is what we call the post-digestive effect. Imagine, if you will: you eat a plateful of healthy-looking grilled veggies complete with mushrooms, spinach, onions, carrots and squash. Later in the week you notice your hands are aching and remember that every now and then you get joint pain.

Maybe the post-digestive effects of mushrooms are causing you pain. How would you even remember that what you ate several days ago is causing the joint pain today? By keeping a food journal, you can see clearly how some foods may be causing your body stress. See the food journal on page 210.

IMPORTANT AYURVEDA PRACTICES

Ayurvedic Food Combining

Have you ever wondered why there are so many digestive aids on the market today? There are myriad remedies for gas, bloating, constipation, diarrhea, heartburn and acidity. TV ads tell us that we can't possibly enjoy a good meal without adding some sort of digestive aid. Indeed, if you suffer from heartburn or gas and bloating, then you are probably familiar with these remedies.

Although it is true that these over-the-counter digestive remedies are everywhere, there is a good reason. Most of these digestive symptoms come from poor food combining. The concept of food combining is not something we spend time on in the West, and it may be quite new to you. When we add two or more foods that do not combine well, we reduce agni (digestive fire). Yes—we are right back to that digestive fire again. Remember, low agni will lead to increased ama (digestive toxins), which creates inflammation . . . and inflammation creates disease.

So take a look at your diet and you will see that you may be eating a number of these incompatible foods. Just note which foods you were combining together before you went on this cleanse.

FOOD TYPE	WHAT IT'S INCOMPATIBLE WITH
Beans	Fruit, cheese, eggs, fish, meat, yogurt
Eggs	Fruit, beans, cheese, fish, kitchari, milk, meat, yogurt
Fruit	As a general rule, fruit should be eaten by itself.
Grains	Fruit, tapioca
Honey	Do not boil or cook with honey. Also incompatible with ghee when used in equal quantities (such as on toast)
Hot drinks	Mangos, cheese, fish, meat, starch, yogurt
Lemon	Cucumbers, milk, tomatoes, yogurt
Melons	Everything! Melons, more than any other fruit, should be eaten by itself.
Milk	Bananas, cherries, melons, sour fruits, yeasted breads, fish, kitchari
Nightshades (potato, tomato, peppers, eggplant)	Melon, cucumber, dairy products
Radishes	Bananas, raisins, milk
Tapioca	Fruit especially bananas, mango, beans, raisins, jaggery
Yogurt	Fruit, cheese, eggs, fish, hot drinks, meat, milk, nightshades

POST-CLEANSE MEAL PLAN

The eating plan for the next 6 days could not be simpler. You will keep Kitchari (page 132) for one meal a day. You will change breakfast and one meal. This is where you can begin to experiment with new recipes and go beyond Kitchari. These four rules will help you stay on track:

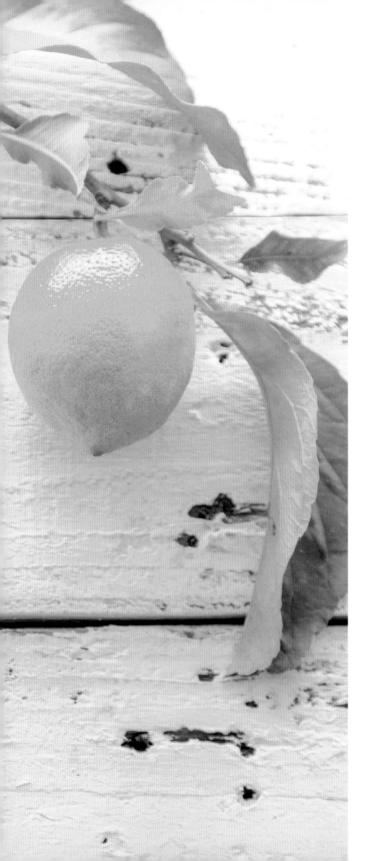

1. Eat a bowl of Kitchari (132) once a day as a meal.

2. Make lunch your heartiest meal of the day. This can mean a bowl of Kitchari with a side of lean protein such as grilled chicken, fish or tofu.

3. Continue to avoid foods that are hard to digest, such as red meat, alcohol, full-fat dairy, flour and sugars, as these will create toxins.

4. Each day when you get up, drink a cup of warm water with a squeeze of lemon and a slice of ginger. This will stimulate your digestive processes and stir your agni. You can make more and sip on this metabolism booster throughout the day.

The Importance of Lemons

High in vitamin C, bioflavonoids and calcium, lemon is alkalizing, which means it:

- Flushes toxins
- Aids digestion and elimination
- Boosts the immune system
- Lowers blood pressure
- Boosts energy
- Improves moods
- Helps with weight loss
- Improves complexion

Shopping List

Follow the sample meal plan and get the ingredients for the meals that you fancy. In addition, you will need:

- 15 lemons
- Ingredients for ojas snack or drinks (pages 158–65)
- Turmeric

POST-CLEANSE RECIPES

Each of the following recipes were designed specifically for the post-cleanse portion of your 25-day cleanse. As with Phases 1 and 2, the recipes were written for Vata with adaptations given for Pitta and Kapha.

Meal Plan for Post-Cleanse

	DAY 20	DAY 21	DAY 22
Breakfast	Ginger Tea (page 63) Scrambled Eggs and Micro Herbs (page 153)	Ginger Tea (page 63) Chia Breakfast Bowl (page 124)	Ginger Tea (page 63) Carrot Muffins with Nut Butter (page 154)
Mid-Morning	Dosha Tea (page 31)		
Lunch	Kitchari (page 132)		
Mid-Afternoon	Ojas-Building Snack (pages 158–65)		
Supper	Cream of Asparagus Soup (page 166)	Cooling Coconut Curry Soup (page 101)	Parsnip and Asparagus Soup (page 169)

	DAY 23	DAY 24	DAY 25
Breakfast	Ginger Tea (page 63) Baked Apples with Dates, Cinnamon and Cardamom (page 127)	Ginger Tea (page 63) Millet Cakes with Nut Butter (page 51)	Ginger Tea (page 63) Savory Spiced Porridge (page 157)
Mid-Morning	Dosha Tea (page 31)		
Lunch	Kitchari (page 132)		
Mid-Afternoon	Ojas-Building Snack (pages 158–65)		
Supper	Winter Farro Salad (page 90)	Baked Tofu with Ginger Rice (page 93)	Chermoula and Pasta (page 82)

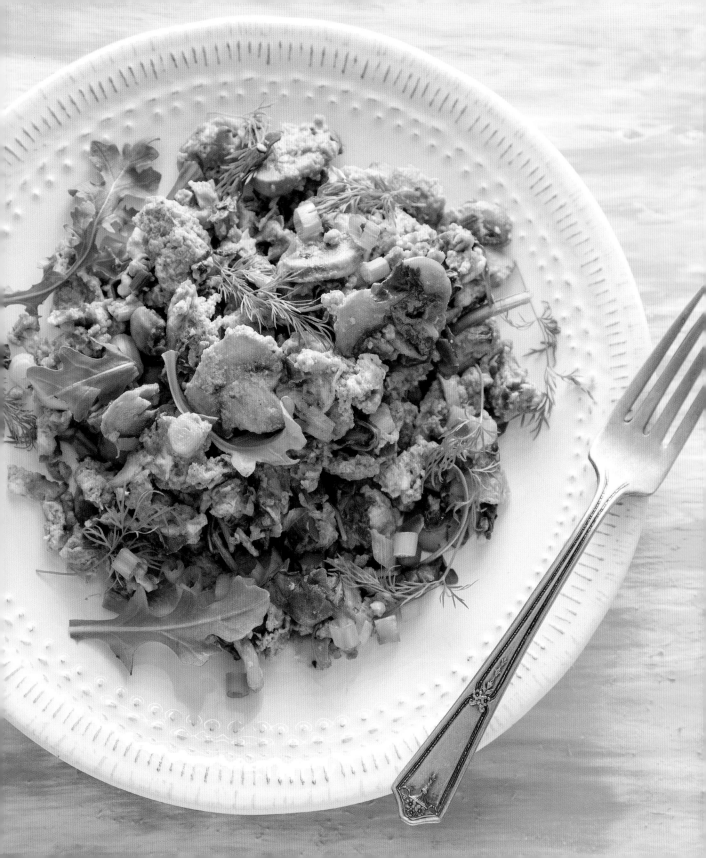

SCRAMBLED EGGS AND MICRO HERBS

This tasty breakfast is protein-rich, and garlic, scallions and chives are antiaging. They also have rasayana properties, which means that they are restorative if you eat them over a long period of time. Scallions are hot, cleansing, nourishing and considered an aphrodisiac. They also kindle the digestive fire, which is great for any sluggish Kapha digestion.

YIELD: 1 serving

3 large eggs

Salt and pepper, as desired

1 tsp ghee

1 tsp cumin powder

½ tsp coriander powder

½ tsp ground turmeric

2 scallions, finely chopped

¾ cup (45 g) sliced mushrooms

Handful of mixed micro herbs (dill, basil, arugula or wheatgrass)

Sprouted wheat bread, toasted, for serving

In a bowl, lightly whisk the eggs and season them with salt and pepper. Set them aside.

Heat the ghee in a skillet. Add the cumin, coriander and turmeric. Sauté for about 1 minute over medium heat. Add the scallions and cook for 1 minute. Add the mushrooms and cook for 1 minute.

Pour the eggs into the skillet. Stir the mixture until it's cooked through. Add the micro herbs and turn off the heat. Serve on a plate and add a slice of sprouted wheat toast.

Dosha Adaptations

RECIPE WRITTEN FOR VATA.
PITTA: Use egg whites only.
KAPHA: Use egg whites. Serve on a bed of spinach and remove the toast.

CARROT MUFFINS WITH NUT BUTTER

Cooked carrots are sweet, nourishing, easy to digest and fibrous. Carrots have a mild pungency that is great for exhaustion and fatigue. They increase your energy, which has earned carrots the titles "tiny ginseng" and the "king of juices." Serve with the nut butter according to your meal plan.

YIELD: 10–12 muffins

1 cup (158 g) brown rice flour

½ tsp baking soda

1 tsp powdered garlic

1 tsp paprika

2 tsp (6 g) dried parsley

¼ tsp salt, plus more as needed

3 eggs

2 cups (220 g) grated carrots

Roasted Saffron Pumpkin Seed Butter (page 51) or Almond and Cashew Nut Butter (page 51), as desired

Preheat the oven to 350°F (180°C). Grease a muffin pan and set it aside.

In a large bowl, mix together the flour, baking soda, garlic, paprika, parsley and salt.

In a small bowl, beat the eggs. Add the eggs to the dry ingredients. Mix well to form a lumpy batter. Add the carrots and gently stir.

Pour the mixture into the muffin tin and bake for 25 to 30 minutes, or until a toothpick inserted into the muffin comes out clean. Serve with the nut butter of your choice.

Dosha Adaptations

RECIPE WRITTEN FOR VATA.
PITTA: Try omitting the garlic and paprika. Add 1 teaspoon of cilantro.
KAPHA: Add 1 teaspoon of red pepper flakes to the batter.

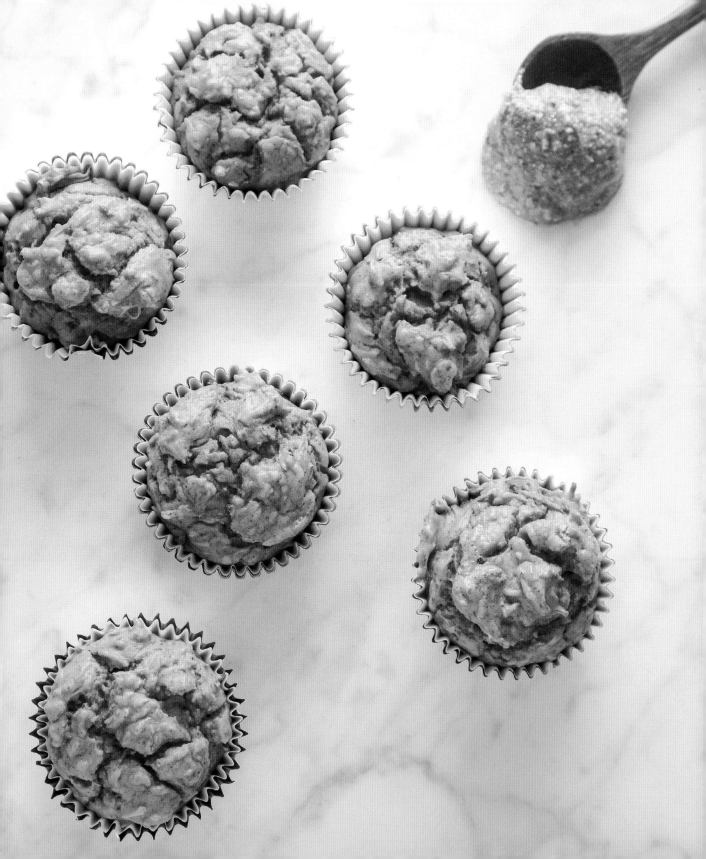

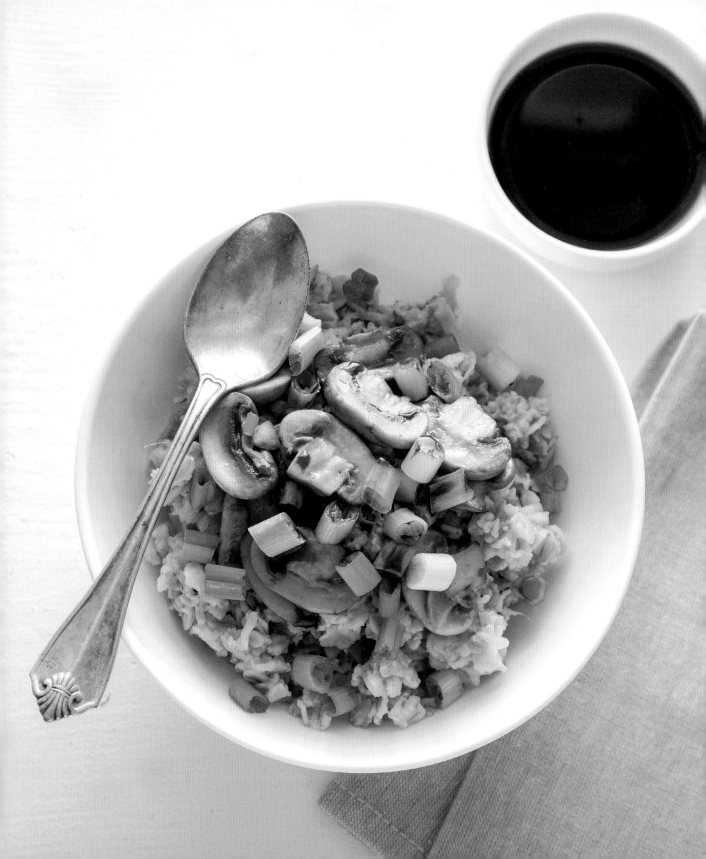

SAVORY SPICED PORRIDGE

Savory spiced porridge is a creamy breakfast grain that has the earthiness of mushrooms combined with delicious spicy flavors. Top it with a dash of soy sauce and scallions and you'll take this simple breakfast to the next level!

YIELD: 2 servings

4 tsp (20 g) ghee, divided

¼ tsp grated ginger

1 cup (100 g) rolled oats

2 cups (480 ml) water, plus more as needed

Salt and pepper, as desired

1 cup (60 g) sliced mushrooms

Dash of soy sauce

Scallions, for garnishing

In a saucepan, heat 1 teaspoon of the ghee and add the ginger. Sauté for 3 minutes, or until fragrant. Add the oats and stir for a few seconds. Add the water, salt and pepper. Bring it to a boil and simmer for 5 to 8 minutes, or until the oats are cooked and you have a thick consistency. Add a little more water if it's too thick. Set it aside.

In a skillet, heat the remaining 3 teaspoons (15 g) ghee and add the mushrooms. Cook over high heat for 3 to 5 minutes, or until the mushrooms are golden brown. Sprinkle with a pinch of salt.

To serve, top the oats with the mushrooms, a dash of soy sauce and the scallions.

Dosha Adaptations

RECIPE WRITTEN FOR VATA.

PITTA: Omit the soy sauce and add chopped mint as a garnish.

KAPHA: Substitute couscous or millet for the oats.

What if there was a special substance in the body that governed aging, immunity, radiant skin, vigor, mood, sleep, digestion, spirituality and physical strength? According to Ayurveda, there is. This substance is called *ojas* (OH-jas). In Sanskrit, ojas means "vitality" or "vigor." It's that glow of health that gives us shiny hair, sparkly eyes, hydrated and glowing skin and most important, sustainable energy.

Ojas is considered the refined by-product of digestion. That means while complete digestion of a meal takes about 24 hours, it takes 30 days for the body to digest food and refine it enough to manufacture ojas (vitality).

Unfortunately, during these 30 days, many factors can compromise its production, and many people have depleted ojas and lack the vigor, immunity, radiant glow and longevity they desire. By adding ojas-building foods, you will feel wonderful with lots of oomph! Try having one ojas-building snack daily while on the post-cleanse.

COCONUT ENERGY BITES

Certain foods help build ojas, and you can enjoy these vitality-building bites anytime you need a pick-me-up.

YIELD: 10–15 small balls

½ **cup (60 g) walnuts**

4 dates, pitted

¼ **cup (20 g) raw carob powder (optional)**

¼ **cup (85 g) maple syrup**

½ **cup (130 g) almond butter**

½ **tsp vanilla extract**

¼ **tsp salt**

½ **cup (70 g) whole almonds**

2 cups (160 g) shredded unsweetened coconut

Place the walnuts in a food processor and pulse until they're coarsely grounded. Add the dates and process until they're well combined. Add the carob powder (if using), maple syrup, almond butter, vanilla and salt. Process until the mixture is thick and smooth. Add the almonds and pulse a few more times until it's well combined.

With your hands, form the mixture into 10 to 15 golf-ball-size balls. Roll the balls in coconut and place them in the fridge until they firm up, about 30 minutes.

Dosha Adaptations

RECIPE WRITTEN FOR VATA.

PITTA: This snack is recommended as a vitality builder for Pittas.

KAPHA: This snack is not recommended due to the sweet taste and rich, heavy qualities of the dates.

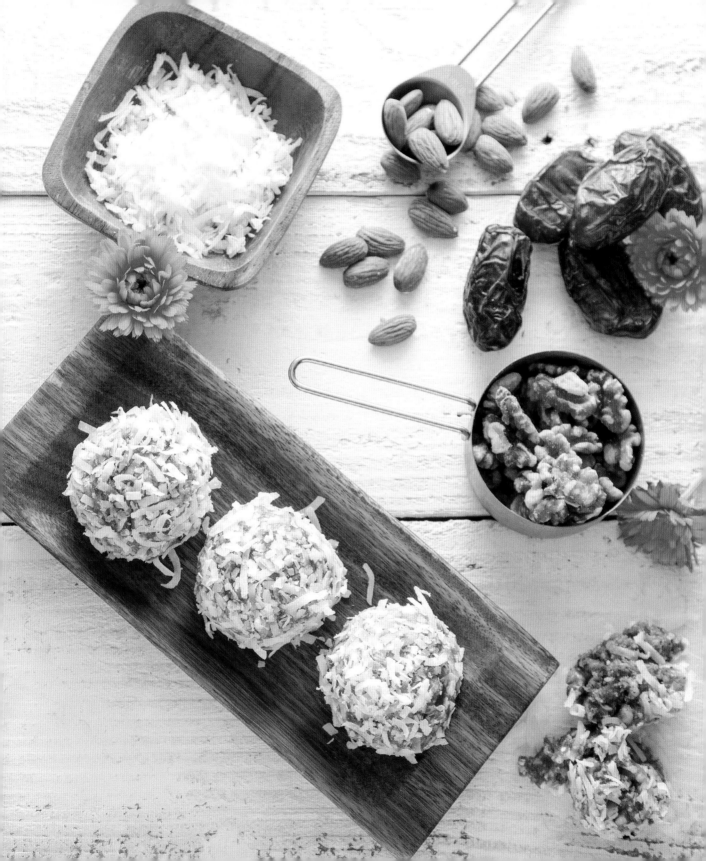

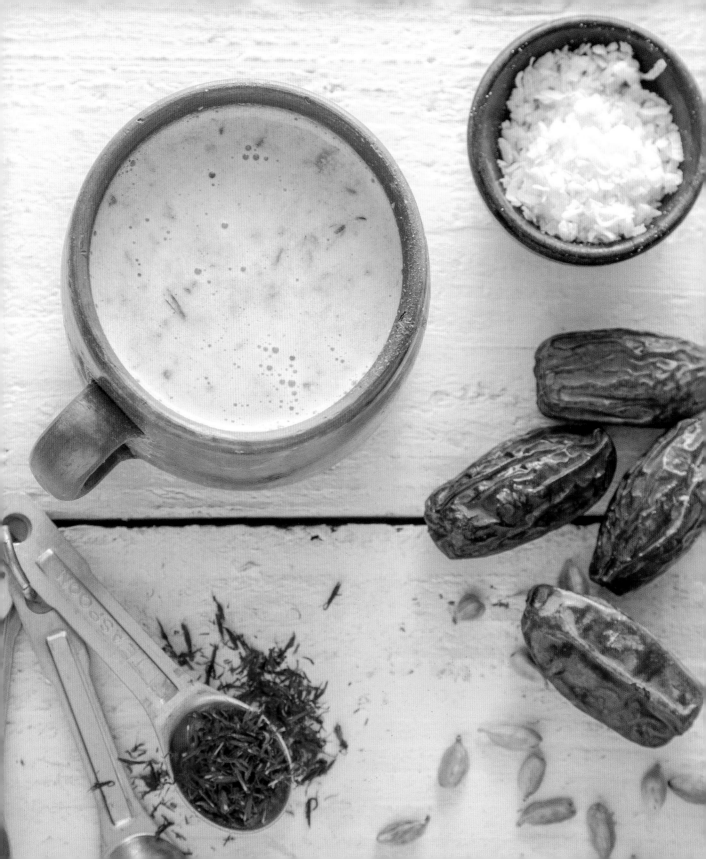

OJAS-BUILDING MILK

Drink this right before bed to boost vitality and support sleep.

YIELD: 1 serving

1 cup (240 ml) milk (non-homogenized cow, almond or coconut)
2 dates, pitted and chopped
4 almonds, chopped
1 tsp coconut flakes
1 tsp ghee
Pinch of saffron
Pinch of cardamom

Place the milk in a small pot. Add the dates, almonds, coconut, ghee, saffron and cardamom to the milk as you slowly bring it to a boil. When it's warm, pour the milk into your favorite mug and drink.

Dosha Adaptations

RECIPE WRITTEN FOR VATA.
PITTA: Use coconut milk.
KAPHA: Not recommended due to the sweet, heavy qualities of coconut and dates.

SWEET LASSI

Ojas builds immunity and vitality, so enjoy this sweet and cooling drink that is a natural probiotic. Goat's milk yogurt is often found in the natural foods section of the grocery store.

YIELD: 2 servings

1½ **cups (360 ml) filtered water**
⅓ **cup (80 g) goat's milk yogurt**
½ **cup (100 g) raw cane sugar**
¼ **tsp ground cardamom**
1 **tbsp (15 ml) rosewater**

In a blender, add the water, yogurt, sugar, cardamom and rosewater. Process until it's smooth and creamy. Pour it into chilled glasses and serve immediately.

Dosha Adaptations

RECIPE WRITTEN FOR VATA.
PITTA: This is a good drink for Pittas. No substitutions needed.
KAPHA: Reduce the sugar to ¼ cup (50 g) and add 1½ teaspoons (4 g) of ground cinnamon.

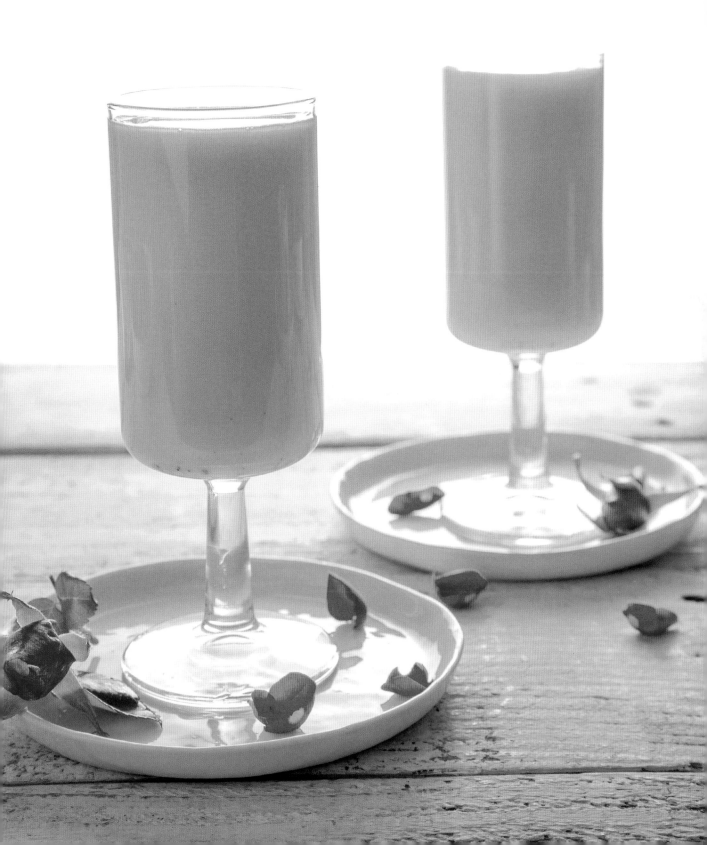

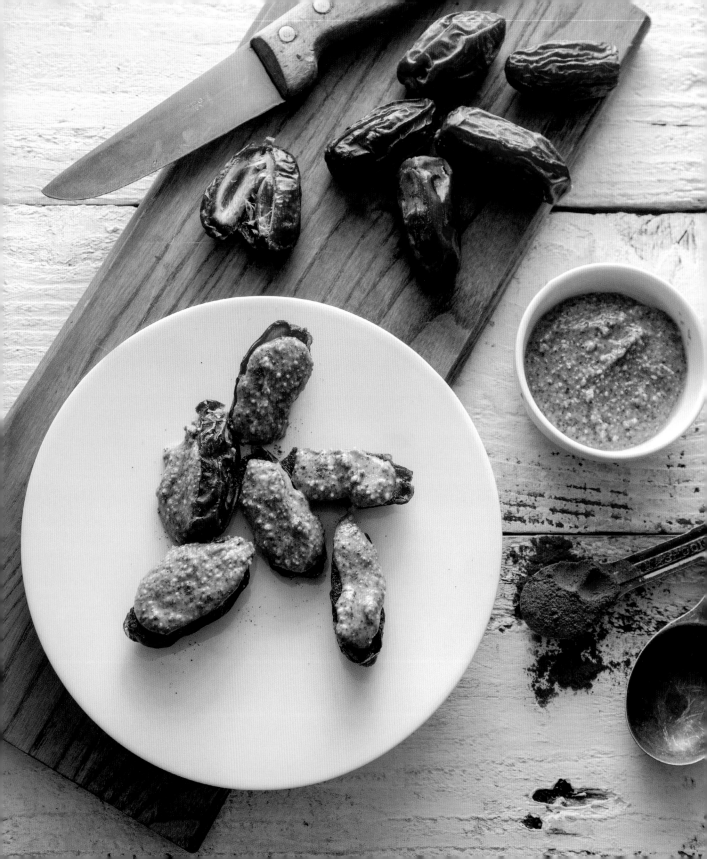

STUFFED DATES

Dates and almonds are considered a healing snack that's excellent for longevity.

YIELD: 4 dates

Pinch of cinnamon
2 tbsp (30 g) almond butter
4 whole dates, pitted

In a small bowl, add the cinnamon and almond butter and stir well. Slice open a date and using a spoon, fill the middle with the almond butter.

Dosha Adaptations

RECIPE WRITTEN FOR VATA.
PITTA: These are a good snack for Pittas. No substitutions needed.
KAPHA: Not recommended due to the sweet, heavy qualities of dates.

CREAM OF ASPARAGUS SOUP

This creamy soup will help carry on the detoxification of the cleanse. A fresh and invigorating flavor with a vivid color, this soup will lighten and brighten as you reintroduce foods back into your everyday diet.

YIELD: 2 servings

1 tbsp (15 g) ghee

2 cloves

½ cinnamon stick

1 bay leaf

1 onion, finely chopped

3 cloves garlic, finely chopped

¼ tsp ginger, finely chopped

1 green chile, seeded and chopped

4 cups (536 g) asparagus, trimmed and cut into small pieces

4 cups (960 ml) vegetable broth or stock

¼ cup (60 ml) coconut milk

Salt and pepper, as desired

Heat the ghee in a saucepan and add the cloves, cinnamon stick and bay leaf. Cook for about 30 seconds. Add the onion, garlic, ginger and chile and sauté for 5 minutes, or until the onion is translucent and just beginning to brown. Add the asparagus and cook for 5 minutes, or until the asparagus begins to soften. Add the vegetable broth and simmer, covered, for 15 minutes.

Remove the pan from the heat and take out the cloves, cinnamon stick and bay leaf and discard them. Allow it to cool slightly and then with either an immersion blender or a blender, process the soup until it's smooth.

Re-warm in a saucepan and add the coconut milk, salt and pepper.

Dosha Adaptations

RECIPE WRITTEN FOR VATA.
PITTA: Reduce the spices by one-half and remove the chile.
KAPHA: Replace the coconut milk with soy milk. Use sunflower oil or corn oil instead of ghee.

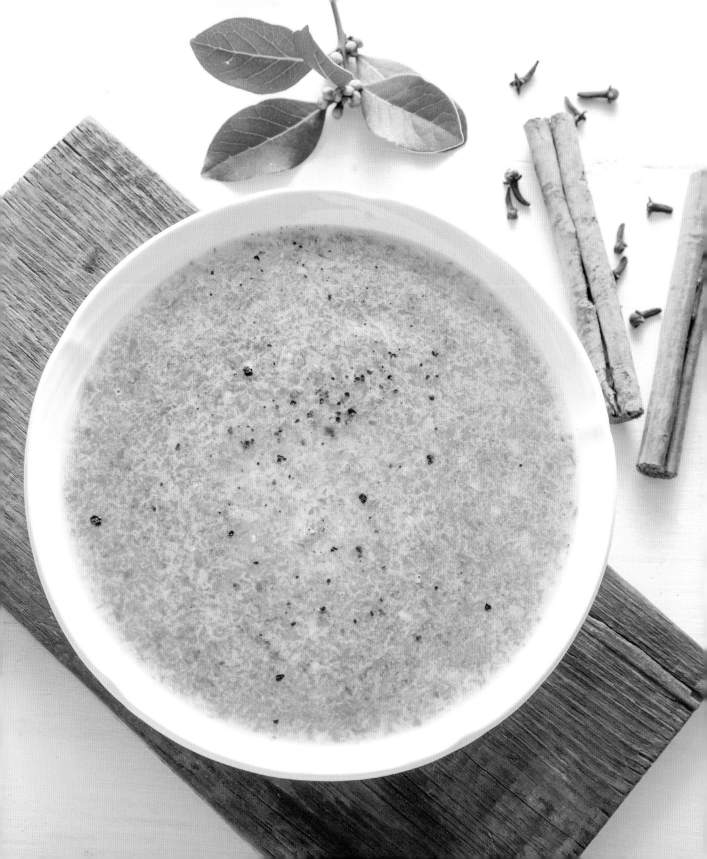

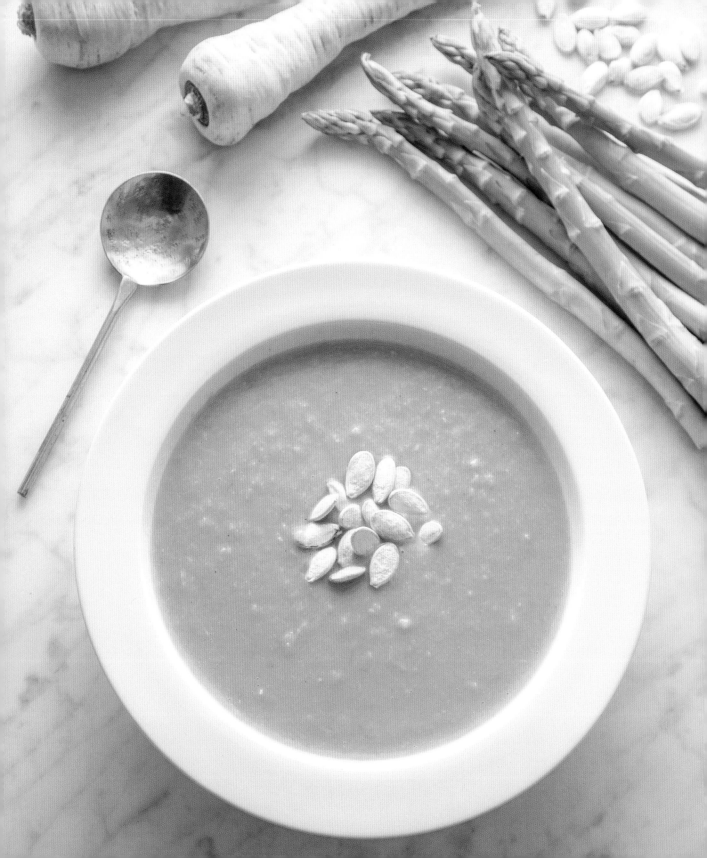

PARSNIP AND ASPARAGUS SOUP

The warm and hearty nature of parsnips promotes sweating, while its bitterness reduces stagnant fluids. Parsnips are perhaps the most satisfying of the "bland" foods. Bland doesn't mean tasteless in Ayurveda, but instead refers to what is known in the West as negative-calorie foods that often have high fiber but a low-calorie content.

YIELD: 4 servings

1 tbsp (15 g) ghee

1 medium white onion, chopped

1 lb (455 g) parsnips, peeled and chopped

1 lb (455 g) asparagus, chopped

4 cups (960 ml) vegetable broth, plus more as needed

Pumpkin seeds, for garnishing

Sea salt and pepper, as desired

In a large saucepan, heat the ghee and add the onion. Sauté for 5 minutes, or until the onion is translucent. Add the parsnips, asparagus and broth. Cook for 15 to 20 minutes, or until the parsnips are very tender.

Puree the mixture in small batches in a blender, until it's smooth. Add more broth to adjust the consistency, as needed. Top with the pumpkin seeds and season with sea salt and pepper.

Dosha Adaptations

RECIPE WRITTEN FOR VATA.

PITTA: Substitute coconut oil for the ghee.

KAPHA: Add 1 tablespoon (9 g) curry powder to the onion as it is cooking.

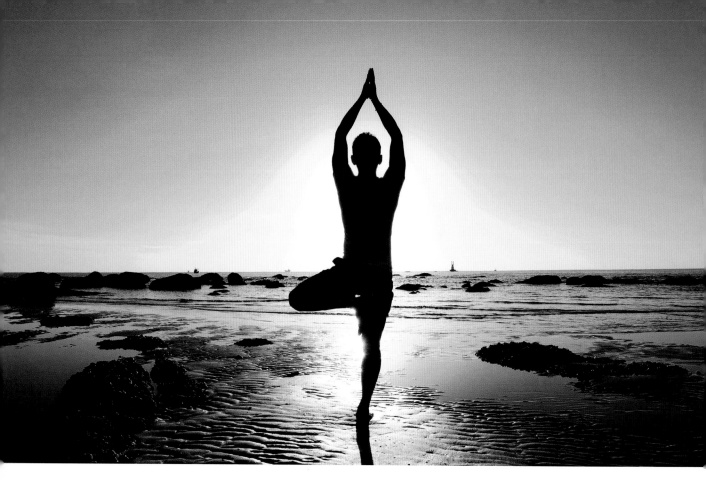

SELF-CARE

Self-care is not selfish, it is sexy. When we spend time on ourselves, we learn to digest our life experiences in a positive way. These practices of yoga, meditation and pranayama will help you discover that you are the power behind your health. You are the author of your life story, and using these practices will help you enjoy the happiest and healthiest life ever. You will become more present, more aware, more in tune and ultimately less stressed. Your body will thank you and your vitality will start flowing naturally.

Energizing Yoga Sequence

This practice is designed to energize and stimulate. Using a series of standing poses, inverted poses and backbends, this practice will have you normalizing your body weight, reducing any congestion and removing excess fluid from the body. The sequence should take about 28 minutes. If you would like to join me with your yoga or meditation, go to www.theholistichighway.com/bookspecial and type in the password "Ayurveda." Here you'll find videos and audio to accompany the book, and we can do this together.

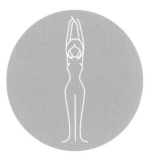

Reach for the Sun (2 minutes)

1. Start in Mountain pose (page 141) with legs together and hands by your side. Inhale as you bring your arms out to the sides and up over your head in a big circular motion. Keep your elbows straight, palms facing each other.

2. On each inhalation, root down through your heels and lift your spine up and back for a slight backbend. Allow your arms to extend you farther.

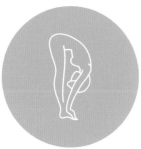

Flop It Forward (1 minute)

1. Exhale as you bend the knees and extend your torso forward and down toward the floor. Extend and straighten your spine.

2. Take 4 breaths here and slowly roll back up to standing to repeat the last pose and this one together again.

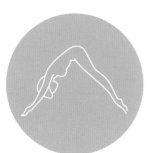

Downward Facing Dog (1 minute)

1. Come into the tabletop position. As you exhale—come onto the balls of your feet and straighten your legs. Keep your heels up as you lengthen the spine, the arms, shoulders and torso.

2. Bring your sitting bones up to the ceiling, making a straight line from hands to tailbone.

3. Holding the straight line, slowly lower your heels to the floor, but only if that works for you. Hold the pose for 4 breaths.

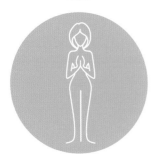

Strong as a Mountain (1 minute)

1. Stand up with your feet parallel and your knees together. Interlace your fingers together so your palms are facing the ceiling.

2. On an inhalation, rise up to the balls of your feet and lift your palms up to the ceiling. Hold for a minute before exhaling and lowering your heels to the floor. Repeat 8 more times.

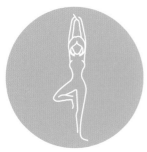

Tree Balance (1 minute)

1. Stand in Mountain Pose. Shift your body weight toward the right foot. Place the ball of your left foot to the right ankle or on the side of the right calf or inner thigh (not beside the right knee). Keep your pelvis square to the front of the room.

2. Bring your hands together in front of your heart or above your head. Breathe comfortably as you balance on one leg. Smile and stay as long as you can. Repeat on the other side.

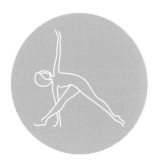

Triangle (2 minutes)

1. Stand with both feet together. Move the left leg approximately 3 to 4 feet (0.9 to 1.2 m) to the side and place the left foot on a forward angle of about 45 degrees.

2. Inhale—raise both arms up to shoulder height. Exhale—shift the weight of your pelvis toward the left as you reach to the side with the torso and right arm (keeping both sides of the torso long and even).

3. Place the right hand on the right leg without collapsing your body weight into it. Look up toward the left hand. Breathe here for 5 full breaths.

4. Inhale—to press into your feet, engage your core and return upright. Exhale—lower your hands to your hips. Inhale—step the left foot forward beside the right foot. Repeat on the second side.

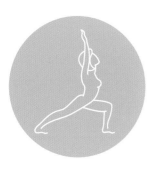

Warrior I (2 minutes)

1. Stand with your legs together and arms by your side. With an exhalation, spread your feet 4 to 5 feet (1.2 to 1.5 m) apart. Inhale and bring your arms straight out to the sides and then up over your head.

2. Turn your right foot and leg 90 degrees out to the left. On an exhale, turn your hips, torso, shoulders and arms to the right facing your right foot. Exhale and bend your right knee until it is over your right heel. Maintain the straight back leg.

3. With each inhalation, bend your knee a little farther. Breathe for 5 breaths here.

4. In your next exhale, straighten the right leg, turn your feet toward the front and bring the back leg forward to meet the front foot. Take a breath here and check in on how you feel. Then, repeat on the other side.

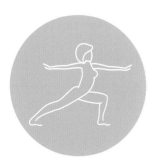

Wild Warrior II (2 minutes)

1. Stand with both feet together. Take the left leg back about 3 to 4 feet (0.9 to 1.2 m). Place the left foot at a 45-degree angle.

2. Raise both arms to shoulder height and as you exhale, bend your right knee until it is in line with your right ankle. Feel the power through your legs. Look over your right hand as if you were a warrior surveying your land in front of you. Stay here for 5 breaths. Inhale to come up and repeat on the other side.

Back Vinyasa (2 minutes)

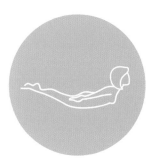

1. Lie facedown on the floor with your legs together and the tops of your feet on the floor.

2. Tighten the backs of your legs. Stretch your arms back along the floor.

3. On your next inhalation, lift your legs, chest, arms and head off the floor. Make sure you look just ahead of you on the floor (no neck strains needed). Take 3 breaths here and slowly lower down. Windshield-wiper the legs side to side. Repeat 4 times.

Ride That Boat (1 minute)

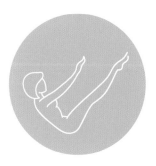

1. Roll onto your back and slowly come to a seated position.

2. Bend the knees and hold the back of the knees. Lean back with a straight spine and straighten the arms.

3. Balancing on the sitting bones, raise your lower legs until they are parallel with the floor.

4. Straighten the legs and let go of the knees, hold the arms and legs parallel with the floor. Inhale and balance. Hold this position for 4 breaths.

5. Bend the knees and bring the legs straight out in front of you.

Stretch It Forward (1 minute)

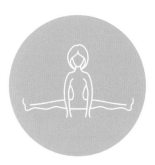

1. Exhale and spread your legs wide with your knees and toes facing the ceiling.

2. Exhale and extend your torso forward while moving your abdomen toward the floor. With each inhalation, lengthen and strengthen the legs. With each exhalation, extend your spine toward your head. Continue for 5 breaths.

3. On the exhale, come back up to a seated position. How do you feel?

Roll It Like an Alligator (2 minutes)

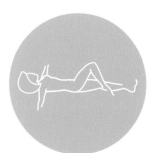

1. Slowly lower yourself back down to the floor with your legs extended and arms in a T-position.

2. Bring your knees into your chest and give them a big hug. Place your arms back into a T-position and slowly lower your knees over to the left while keeping your shoulders flat on the floor.

3. Gently move your head to the right, completing the twist. Stay here for 8 breaths. Inhale and move your knees back to center and repeat on the other side.

Save-It Savasana (10 minutes)

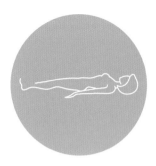

1. Lie down comfortably on your back with your legs extended. Cover yourself with a blanket if you are apt to get cold.

2. Pull the shoulders down and back as you lengthen your arms along your side, palms up. Lengthen your neck. Inhale deeply, exhale and allow your whole body to relax.

3. Systematically relax each part of your body beginning with your feet. Relax your toes, then ankles, then calves, knees and hips, all while moving your awareness up through your body, consciously relaxing any stress or tight spots along the way. Keep your breath deep and natural and allow yourself to surrender into the stillness of this pose.

4. After about 10 minutes, slowly deepen your breath, wiggle your fingers and toes, bring some movement back into your body by stretching in any way that feels good to you.

5. Roll onto your right side, stay there for a couple of minutes and then use your hands to push yourself into an upright seated position.

Knowing Your Place Meditation

If you would like to join me with your yoga or meditation, go to www.theholistichighway.com/bookspecial and type in the password "Ayurveda." Here you'll find videos and audio to accompany the book, and we can do this together.

Look around at all that lives, at all that *is*. See how connected we all are to the workings of the universe. From the tiniest wildflower to the tallest redwood in the forest, each creation contains its own energy and so it is with us.

We are intricately connected to the world. We receive energy, life-sustaining nourishment and support from the world around us. But inside each of us is our own source of love, joy and wisdom. Our ability to love, live, feel and be happy comes from our own hearts.

Look inside yourself. Feel your vitality and energy. Feel your essence. It is pure love. Everything you need to live and love is within you. Nurture yourself. Let yourself grow. Learn to grow and walk in the ways of love. Learn from all who cross your path. Value your connections to others and the world around you. Receive and give freely as you walk down the road.

Pranayama: Three-Part Belly Breath

As you learn this deep breath—feel how your mind slows, your breath deepens and you automatically start relaxing. Lie on the floor in a comfortable position or you can also do this seated in a chair if that is more comfortable.

1. Place one hand on your belly and the other over your heart. Take a couple of breaths to connect to those two points.

2. On the inhale, take the breath into your belly as if you were filling up a vase with water. Then take that breath up through the ribs and into the chest. Hold it at the chest for just a moment. And then exhale, taking the breath from the chest to the ribs and back to the belly, bringing the belly button in toward your back. Repeat this three-part breath for 5 minutes.

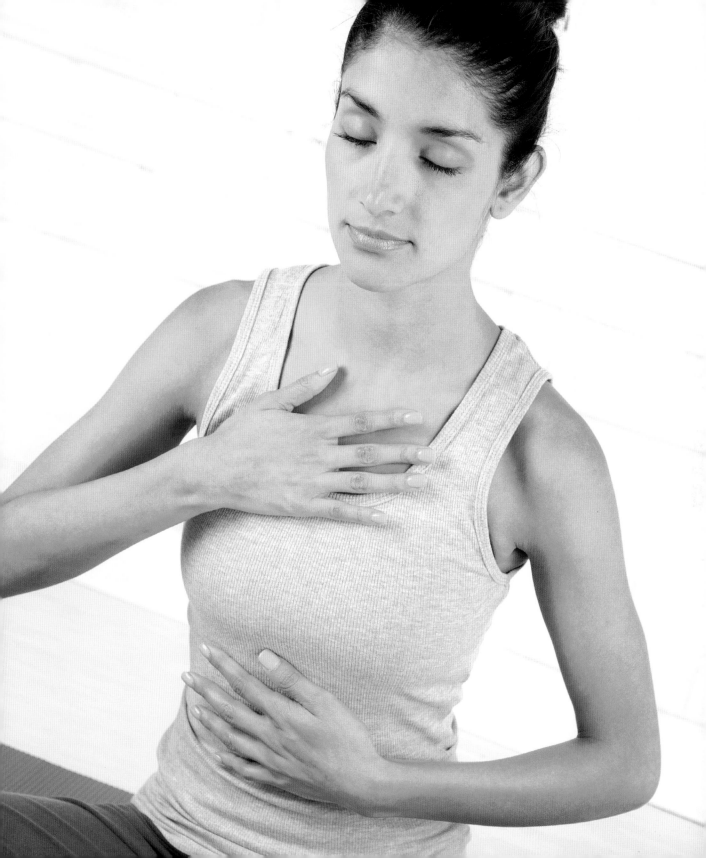

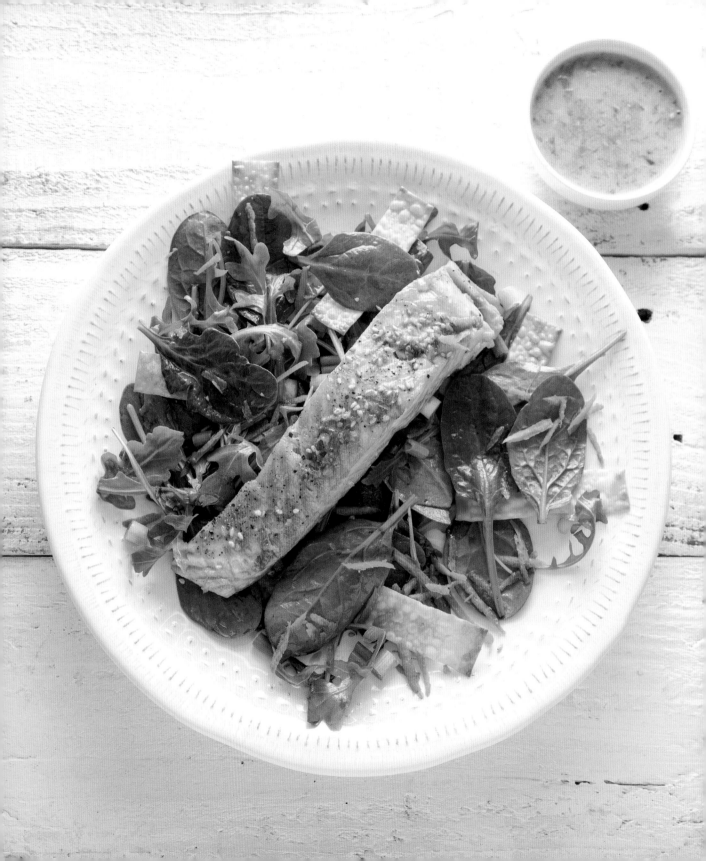

Chapter 5

AYURVEDA LIVING FOR THE REST OF YOUR LIFE

Wow—you've done it! You have completed the Ayurveda cleanse and you are probably feeling quite differently now that you have come off the post-cleanse and have spent the last 25 days eating foods that have ignited your agni (digestive fire) and reduced ama (toxins). Think back to when you started. Have you lost some weight? Do you have more energy and feel more stable—a little lighter? Hopefully, the answers are yes! This chapter spends some time on the next steps: how to live and thrive as you go forward.

EATING FOR YOUR DOSHA

Now that you have completed the cleanse and know your dosha, you can take a much more individualized approach to your food and further tweak your journey to great health and vitality. Use your dosha as a guide and trust your intuition. I am always amazed when a client going over their meal plan tells me, "Oh, I always wanted to eat that, but I thought it wasn't healthy for me." For instance, if you are a Vata suffering through salads because you think it's healthy but are craving warm soups and stews, you can now trust that intuition.

The best way to truly know your dosha is to see an Ayurveda practitioner. Dosha quizzes are a lot of fun and they certainly give some valuable information; however, all quizzes (including mine) are limited in

two major areas. First, quizzes are a snapshot, a single moment in history, and they can only spit back the information you put in. Second, they are self-reporting. You put down who you think you are—and that is not necessarily who you are. It is important to go deeper into your bio-individuality and explore all aspects that make up you. In the Holistic Highway Programs, we include genetic testing as well, so we can get to know you right down to the molecular level. This information is then combined with the information from an Ayurveda consultation to create a comprehensive wellness plan that meets your specific health needs. Are you eating the right foods in the right seasons? Are you getting up at the right time and going to bed at the right time? Are you doing the right exercises to get the best results for your particular dosha?

As you are already aware by now, Ayurveda endorses a balanced diet that nurtures not only the body but also the mind, senses and spirit. Food, after all, is a source of energy and strength.

Take a look at the following 5-day meal plans for each dosha. These are easy and delicious dinner recipes as you start adding foods back that are right for you. Each meal plan includes a shopping list, so you can get the right food over the weekend and know you are eating all the right foods for you throughout the week.

SAMPLE VATA MEAL PLAN AND RECIPES

Shopping List

Meat and Seafood

- 2 boneless, skinless chicken breasts
- 4 salmon fillets

Vegetables and Fruit

- 1 small bunch asparagus
- 5 oz (140 g) carrots
- 3 celery ribs
- 1 cucumber
- 1" (2.5-cm) piece ginger
- 2 scallions
- 3 lemons
- 1 (10-oz [280-g]) bag mixed greens
- ½ cup (120 ml) orange juice
- 2 bunches fresh parsley
- 2 large portobello mushrooms
- 2 red onions
- 4½ oz (130 g) strawberries
- 2 sweet red peppers
- 1 tomato

Bakery and Miscellaneous

- 4 kaiser rolls
- 2 tbsp (30 g) pesto
- 7 oz (200 g) quinoa
- 2 whole-wheat tortillas
- 4 wonton wrappers

Dairy

- 1 tbsp (15 g) light yogurt
- 1 tbsp (15 g) light sour cream
- 2 tbsp (10 g) shredded mozzarella cheese

Pantry Staples

You may have these in your pantry, but if not, this is what you will need each week.

- Adzuki beans (red beans)
- Almond butter
- Almonds
- Avocados
- Balsamic vinegar
- Basil (fresh)
- Basmati rice
- Black pepper
- Butter
- Cardamom
- Cayenne
- Chicken broth or stock
- Chili powder
- Cilantro (fresh)
- Coriander
- Cumin
- Fennel
- Garlic
- Ginger (fresh)
- Honey
- Kosher salt
- Mango chutney
- Maple syrup
- Milk
- Mint (fresh)
- Mustard
- Olive oil and olive oil spray
- Oregano
- Pine nuts
- Rice noodles
- Sesame oil
- Sesame seeds
- Soy sauce
- Turmeric
- Vegetable broth or stock
- Vinegar

SESAME GINGER SALMON SALAD FOR MONDAY

This meal, using the ojas-building qualities of salmon and the grounding, calming qualities of sesame, is a rejuvenating meal. With the added health benefits of ginger, this meal is a really nourishing choice that will have you feeling calm, grounded and energized.

YIELD: 2–4 servings

FOR THE GINGER SESAME DRESSING

2 tbsp (30 ml) soy sauce

1" (2.5-cm) piece ginger, chopped

1 clove garlic, chopped

2 tbsp (6 g) scallions

1 tbsp (10 g) sesame seeds

¼ cup (60 ml) extra-virgin olive oil

3 tbsp (45 ml) white vinegar

2 tbsp (40 g) maple syrup

1 tbsp (15 ml) sesame oil, plus more as needed

FOR THE WONTON STRIPS

4 wonton wrappers, cut into ½" (12-mm) strips

Sesame oil, as desired

Salt and pepper, as desired

FOR THE SALMON

4 (4-oz [115-g]) salmon pieces

Salt and pepper, as desired

1 tbsp (15 ml) extra-virgin olive oil

FOR SERVING

1 cup (20 g) mixed greens

1 cup (128 g) shredded carrots

Scallions, for garnishing

Preheat the oven to 475°F (240°C).

To make the ginger sesame dressing, add the soy sauce, ginger, garlic, scallions, sesame seeds, olive oil, vinegar, maple syrup and sesame oil in a food processor. Pulse and blend until smooth. Keep it in the refrigerator until you're ready to serve.

To make the wonton strips, on a rimmed baking pan, toss the wonton wrappers with a drizzle of sesame oil, and then season them with salt and pepper. Spread the strips in an even layer across the pan and bake for 4 minutes, or until golden brown.

To make the salmon, season the salmon with salt and pepper. Heat a cast-iron skillet over high heat and add the olive oil. When the pan is almost smoking, carefully place the salmon in the pan skin-side up. Cook for 4 minutes on each side.

To serve, toss the mixed greens and carrots in a bowl with most of the ginger sesame dressing. Serve each piece of the salmon on a bed of greens, garnish them with scallions and the wonton strips and drizzle with the remaining dressing.

See image on page 176.

Dosha Adaptations

PITTA: Remove the garlic and add 1 teaspoon of cilantro.
KAPHA: No substitutions needed.

QUINOA ASPARAGUS PILAF
FOR TUESDAY

Quinoa is a seed that provides an excellent source of protein. Easy to prepare, easy to digest and nutrient-dense, quinoa is a simple, practical and straightforward choice. Asparagus is a rejuvenative vegetable, especially for women.

YIELD: 2-4 servings

2 cups (480 ml) chicken or vegetable stock

1 cup (180 g) quinoa, rinsed

1-2 tbsp (15-30 ml) extra-virgin olive oil, plus extra as needed

½ red onion, finely sliced into rings

3 celery ribs, sliced

1 small bunch asparagus, sliced

1½ tsp (4 g) cumin

Pinch of cayenne

1 tsp lemon zest

½ cup (60 g) chopped toasted almonds

Juice of 1 lemon

½ cup (30 g) chopped parsley

In a medium saucepan, bring the stock to a boil. Add the quinoa, reduce the heat, cover and cook for 15 minutes, or per the quinoa package instructions. The quinoa should absorb all the broth. Remove the pan from the heat, fluff the quinoa with a fork, cover and let it stand for 15 minutes.

In a medium saucepan, heat the olive oil and sauté the onion rings for 5 minutes, or until the onion is limp and starting to caramelize. Be careful not to burn the onion. Add the celery and asparagus and sauté for 4 minutes, or until the asparagus is crispy but cooked. Add the cumin, cayenne and lemon zest, stir and cook for 1 minute. Remove the pan from the heat.

In a large bowl, toss the quinoa, sautéed vegetables, almonds and lemon juice together. Finish with a splash of the olive oil and the parsley.

Dosha Adaptations

PITTA: Omit the cayenne and add cilantro or mint instead of parsley.
KAPHA: Remove the nuts and replace them with pumpkin seeds.

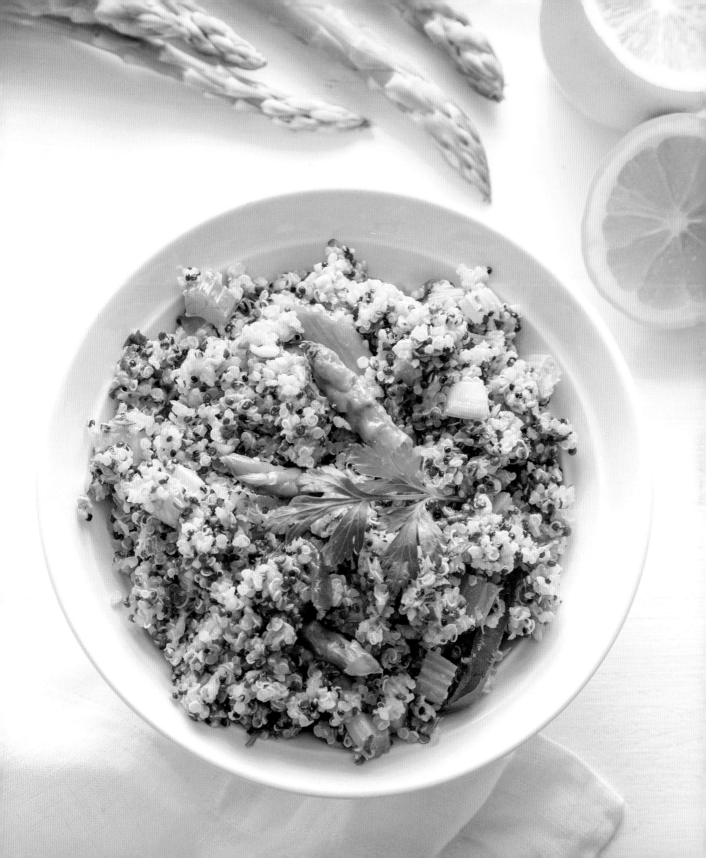

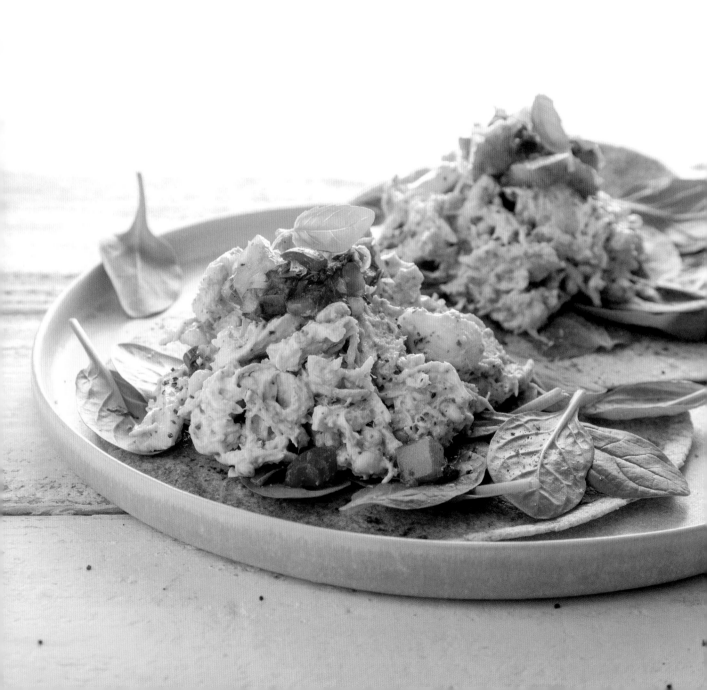

BRUSCHETTA CHICKEN PESTO WRAPS
FOR WEDNESDAY

Basil is balancing for Vatas and is used to maintain and promote the long-term health of the respiratory tract. It is also used to settle stomach disorders and to enhance digestion. A mild natural sleep aid, basil enhances the quality of sleep, which is so important for anyone with Vata in them.

YIELD: 2 servings

1 tomato, diced, with seeds removed

1 tbsp (10 g) minced onion

1–2 tbsp (3–6 g) minced fresh basil or 1 tsp dry basil

1 tsp balsamic vinegar

Salt and pepper, as desired

1 tbsp (15 g) light yogurt

1 tbsp (15 g) light sour cream or plain Greek yogurt

2 tbsp (30 g) pesto

1 tsp fresh lemon juice

Zest of ½ lemon

5 oz (140 g) shredded or diced cooked chicken breast

1 tbsp (10 g) toasted pine nuts

½ cup (24 g) shredded romaine lettuce or spinach leaves

2 wheat tortillas

In a medium bowl, combine the tomato, onion, basil, balsamic vinegar, salt and pepper. Set it aside.

In a medium bowl, combine the yogurt, sour cream, pesto, lemon juice and zest. Stir the mixture and combine it with the chicken and pine nuts, stirring until they're combined.

Layer the lettuce on the tortillas, top with the chicken mixture and then add the bruschetta mixture.

Dosha Adaptations

PITTA: Remove the pine nuts and use sunflower seeds.
KAPHA: Add ½ teaspoon of red pepper flakes and use almond cream or soy yogurt instead of yogurt. Use corn tortillas.

GRILLED VEGETABLE SANDWICHES WITH CILANTRO PESTO
FOR THURSDAY

There is so much that benefits you in this meal, from the earthy grounding qualities of mushrooms, to the cooling qualities of cilantro. We also added some parsley as a natural detoxifier and the protein of the pine nuts makes this meal a healthy choice.

YIELD: 4 sandwiches

FOR THE PESTO

1 cup (20 g) packed fresh cilantro sprigs

¼ cup (10 g) packed fresh parsley sprigs

2 tbsp (10 g) grated Parmesan cheese

2 cloves garlic, peeled

2 tbsp (30 ml) water

1 tbsp (10 g) pine nuts

1 tbsp (15 ml) extra-virgin olive oil

FOR THE SANDWICHES

2 large sweet red peppers

4 thick slices portobello mushrooms

Olive oil spray

Salt and pepper, as desired

½ cup (56 g) shredded part-skim mozzarella cheese

4 kaiser rolls, split

To make the pesto, place the cilantro, parsley, Parmesan cheese and garlic in a food processor and pulse until they're chopped. Add the water and pine nuts and process until it's blended. While processing, slowly add the oil.

To make the sandwiches, grill the peppers, covered, over medium heat for 10 to 15 minutes, or until the skins are blistered and blackened. Immediately place the peppers in a large bowl and let them stand, covered, for 20 minutes. Peel off and discard the charred skin. Cut the peppers in half and remove the stems and seeds.

Lightly spritz both sides of the mushroom slices with the oil spray and sprinkle with salt and pepper. Grill, covered, over medium heat for 3 to 5 minutes on each side, or until tender. Top with the peppers and sprinkle with the mozzarella cheese. Grill, covered, for 2 to 3 minutes, or until the cheese is melted. Remove them from the grill.

Spread the kaiser rolls with the pesto, place the mushrooms and peppers in the rolls and top with more pesto.

Dosha Adaptations

PITTA: Remove the pine nuts and use sunflower seeds. Use goat cheese instead of Parmesan.
KAPHA: Use goat cheese as the cheese.

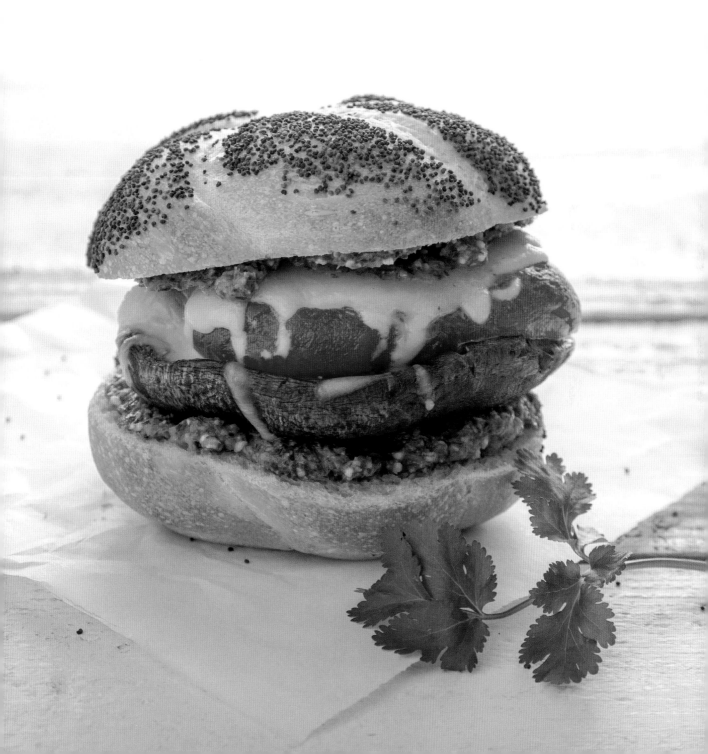

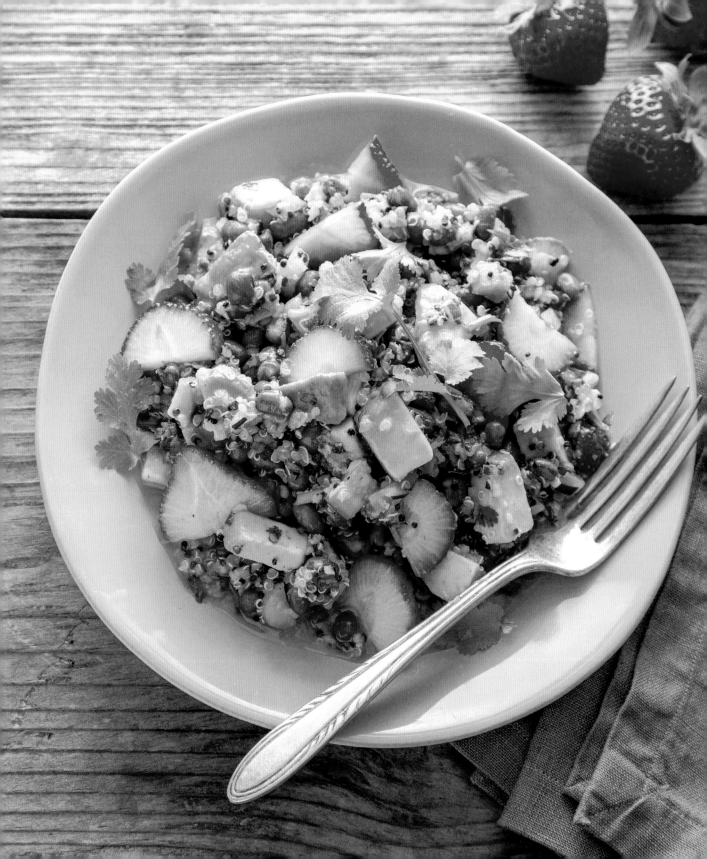

CITRUS STRAWBERRY QUINOA SALAD
FOR FRIDAY

We have put together lots of rejuvenative foods in this salad that are designed to balance Vata, including quinoa, adzuki beans and avocado. Add that to the sweet citrus . . . and Vatas are happy and gas-free!

YIELD: 4–6 servings

FOR THE DRESSING

½ cup (120 ml) freshly squeezed orange juice

1½ tbsp (23 ml) freshly squeezed lemon juice

2–3 tsp (14–20 g) honey

2 tbsp (30 ml) extra-virgin olive oil

½ heaping tsp kosher salt

A few cracks of freshly ground black pepper

1 clove garlic, minced

FOR THE SALAD

1 cup (180 g) quinoa

2 cups (480 ml) water or chicken (or vegetable) broth

½ medium cucumber, peeled, seeded and diced

½ medium red onion, minced

¼ cup (10 g) fresh minced cilantro or parsley

1 cup (140 g) strawberries, sliced

1 (15-oz [430-g]) can adzuki beans, rinsed and drained

1–2 avocados, cut into small cubes

Salt and pepper, as desired

For the dressing, in a bowl, whisk together the orange juice, lemon juice, honey, olive oil, salt, pepper and garlic. Set this aside.

For the salad, cook the quinoa in the water or broth according to the package directions.

In a large salad bowl, combine the cucumber, onion, cilantro, strawberries and adzuki beans. Toss them with the quinoa.

Drizzle the dressing over the mixture and toss to combine it. Before serving, add the avocados and season it with salt and pepper.

Dosha Adaptations

PITTA: Remove the garlic and use cilantro instead of parsley.

KAPHA: Substitute chickpeas for adzuki beans. Omit the avocado and use sunflower oil instead of olive oil.

SAMPLE PITTA MEAL PLAN AND RECIPES

Shopping List

Meat and Seafood

- 1–2 chicken breasts
- 4 chicken legs with thighs
- ¼ lb (115 g) turkey sausage

Vegetables and Fruit

- 2 acorn squashes
- ½ tbsp (2 g) basil
- 2 carrots
- 2 celery ribs
- 6 cloves garlic
- 1 gold potato
- 1 cup (20 g) mixed greens
- 1½ cups (224 g) diced green bell peppers
- 1½ cups (100 g) kale
- 8 oz (230 g) frozen mango
- ¼ cup (30 g) peas
- ½ cup (70 g) raisins
- 1 russet potato
- 1 Spanish onion
- 1 cup (100 g) diced seasonal squash
- 1 sweet potato

Bakery and Miscellaneous

- 1 cup (125 g) all-purpose flour
- 2 tsp (7 g) arrowroot starch
- ½ cup (120 g) coconut cream
- 2 small bunches dill
- 1 tbsp (3 g) fresh mint
- 4 oz (115 g) egg noodles
- ⅛ tsp garam masala
- ½ tsp paprika
- 1 tbsp (15 ml) red wine vinegar
- 2 tsp (10 ml) sesame oil

Pantry Staples

You may have these in your pantry, but if not, this is what you will need each week.

- Almonds
- Barley
- Basmati rice
- Black beans
- Black pepper
- Cardamom
- Chicken broth
- Coconut flakes
- Coconut milk
- Coconut oil
- Coriander
- Cumin
- Fennel
- Ghee
- Ginger
- Himalayan mineral salt
- Lentils
- Maple syrup
- Mint
- Olive oil
- Sunflower oil
- Sunflower seeds
- Turmeric
- Unsalted butter
- Vegetable broth

CHICKEN NOODLE SOUP WITH DILL
AND FENNEL FOR MONDAY

We like the detoxification of celery along with the cooling qualities of fennel. Combine that with the protein of chicken and this is an excellent meal for you Pittas, especially in fall.

YIELD: 2 servings

2 bone-in chicken thighs and legs

3 cups (720 ml) water

2 carrots, diced

1 large Spanish onion, diced

3 cloves garlic, minced

2 celery ribs, diced

1 fennel bulb, diced

2 tbsp (30 ml) chicken broth

4 oz (115 g) egg noodles

Salt and pepper, as desired

1 bunch dill, chopped

Place the chicken pieces and water in a large pot. Cover and heat to boiling over high heat. Add the carrots, onion, garlic, celery, fennel and chicken broth to the pot and return to a boil, covered. Once the soup boils, uncover and reduce the heat to medium. Simmer for 20 minutes, or until the chicken is cooked through. Use a spoon to skim off any foam.

Remove the chicken from the pot. When it's just cool enough to handle, remove the meat from the bones and chop or shred it into bite-size pieces. Discard the skin and bones.

Add the noodles to the pot. Simmer for 4 minutes, and then add the chicken meat. Cook for 2 to 5 minutes, or until the noodles are cooked. Season the broth with salt and pepper, to taste. Just before serving, add most of the dill to the pot. Divide the soup between two bowls. Garnish each bowl with the remaining dill.

Dosha Adaptations

VATA: This is also a good meal for Vatas. Serve with some warmed bread and ghee.
KAPHA: Switch out the egg noodles for a corn pasta or rice.

SAVORY STIR-FRY FOR TUESDAY

Kale has bitter and astringent qualities that help to detox and lighten the body. This is really good for Pittas when they need to remove excess heat.

YIELD: 4 servings

1 tbsp (15 ml) red wine vinegar

1 tbsp (20 g) maple syrup

2 tsp (10 g) coconut oil

2 tsp (7 g) arrowroot starch

2 tbsp (30 ml) extra-virgin olive oil

1 cup (100 g) seasonal squash, peeled and diced

1½ cups (224 g) diced green bell pepper

½ cup (34 g) chopped kale

2 cloves garlic, minced

2 tsp (6 g) cardamom

1 tsp minced fresh ginger

3 cups (420 g) shredded cooked chicken

½ cup (70 g) raisins

Cooked basmati rice, as desired

In a bowl, whisk together the red wine vinegar, maple syrup, coconut oil and arrowroot. Set it aside.

In a large skillet or wok, heat the olive oil over medium-high heat and add the squash. Stir-fry until the squash begins to brown slightly. Add the green pepper and sauté until it begins to soften, 4 to 5 minutes. Add the kale, garlic, cardamom and ginger and cook until the kale begins to wilt, 5 to 6 minutes. Add the chicken and raisins to the skillet and heat for 2 minutes.

Slowly add the sauce to the skillet or wok. Cook for 5 minutes, or until all the vegetables are tender. Remove the skillet from the heat and allow it to cool for 5 minutes. Serve over rice, if desired.

Dosha Adaptations

VATA: Add a pinch of nutmeg.
KAPHA: Use cranberries instead of raisins. Use ½ tablespoon (8 g) of sugar instead of the maple syrup.

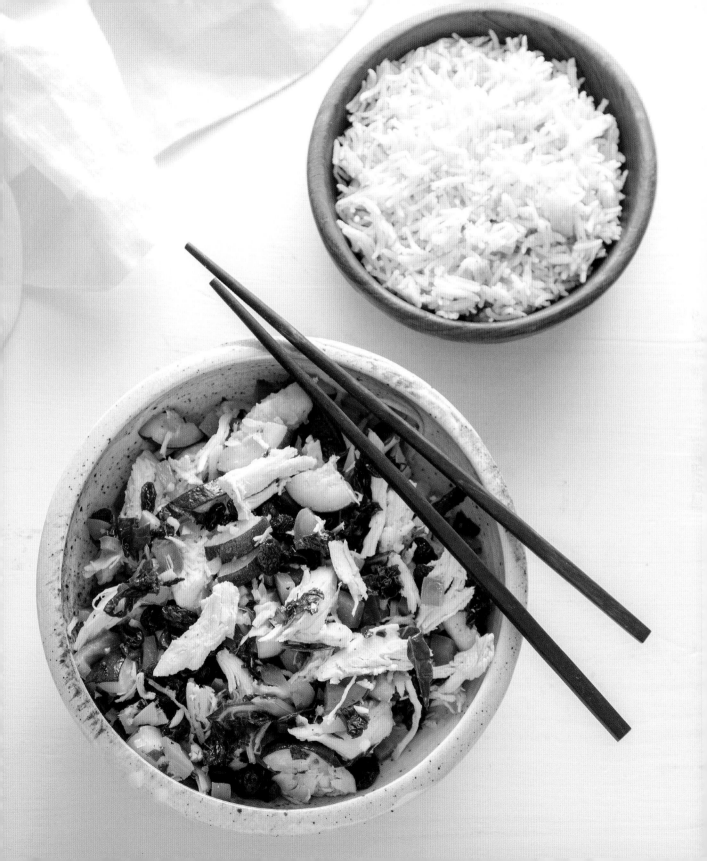

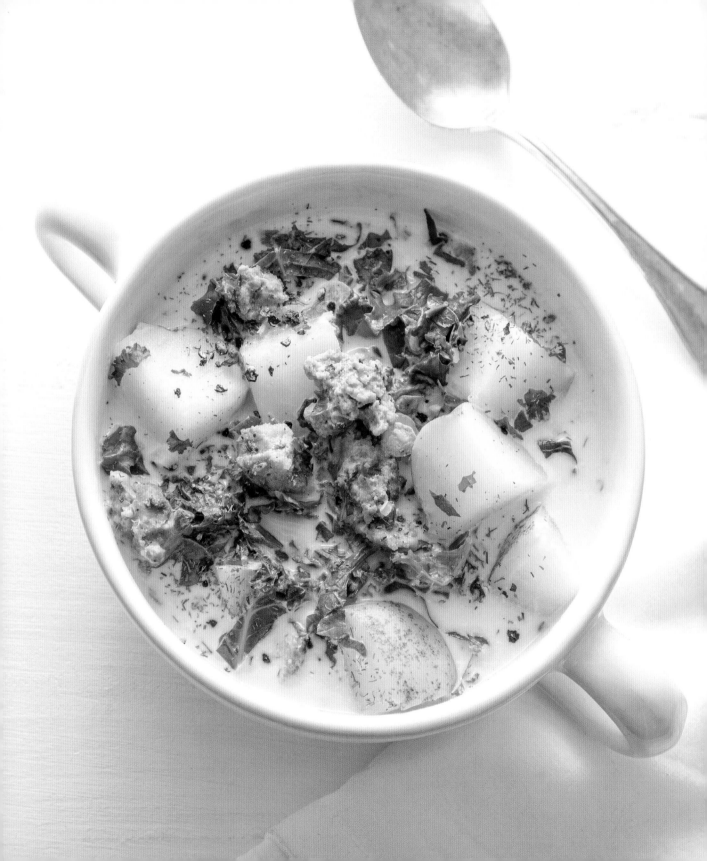

ZUPPA TOSCANA FOR WEDNESDAY

Dill has been used for culinary and medicinal purposes for hundreds of years. It has excellent carminative properties, which means it soothes the digestive system and is used in Ayurveda for the treatment of ulcers, fever, cardiac problems, bronchitis, syphilis and menstrual disorders.

YIELD: 3 servings

2 tsp (10 ml) extra-virgin olive oil

4 oz (115 g) turkey sausage

1 clove garlic, minced

1 tsp dried dill

3 cups (720 ml) chicken broth or stock

1 large russet potato, cut into 1½" (4-cm) chunks

½ cup (120 g) coconut cream

Pepper, as desired

1 cup (60 g) roughly chopped kale, spinach, collard greens or swiss chard

In large saucepan, heat the oil. Add the turkey sausage and sauté over medium heat for 5 minutes, or until the sausage has cooked through. Remove the sausage from the pan with a slotted spoon and set it aside. Stir in the garlic and dill. Cook for 3 minutes. Drain away the excess drippings.

Pour in the chicken broth and bring the liquid to a boil. Once boiling, add the potato and cook for 15 minutes, or until the potatoes are softened. Stir in the coconut cream and cooked sausage. Cook for 8 minutes, or until heated through. Add pepper to taste and stir in the chopped greens just before serving.

Dosha Adaptations

VATA: Use almond milk instead of the coconut cream.

KAPHA: Use almond milk instead of the coconut cream and add a pinch of red pepper flakes.

ACORN SQUASH BISQUE
FOR THURSDAY

Acorn squash is a nourishing, grounding vegetable with a nice touch of sweetness, which can be the centerpiece of any hearty meal. Acorn squash by itself dries out the mouth; therefore it can dry out your intestinal tract too. Great for Pittas who tend toward loose stools.

YIELD: 4 servings

2 acorn squashes

1 tbsp (15 g) ghee

Salt and pepper, as desired

½ tsp fresh dill, plus more for garnishing

1 (14.5-oz [435-ml]) carton vegetable broth

2 cups (480 ml) water, plus more as needed

½ cup (120 ml) coconut milk

Place the squashes on a paper towel and microwave on high for 8 to 10 minutes, or until just tender when pierced with the tip of a paring knife. Remove them from the microwave and halve each squash lengthwise. When cool enough to handle, scoop out and discard the seeds. Scrape out the flesh into a bowl and discard the skin.

In a large saucepan, heat the ghee over medium heat. Add the squash and season with salt and pepper. Cook, stirring occasionally, for 3 to 5 minutes, or until tender. Add the dill, broth and water. Bring it to a boil over high heat, reduce to medium heat and cook for 10 to 12 minutes, or until the squash is very tender.

Working in batches, puree the mixture in a blender until it's very smooth. Return the mixture to the saucepan, add the coconut milk and season generously with salt and pepper. Thin the bisque, if needed, by adding more water. Serve garnished with dill.

Dosha Adaptations

VATA: Use a light cream instead of coconut milk.
KAPHA: Use soy milk instead of coconut milk.

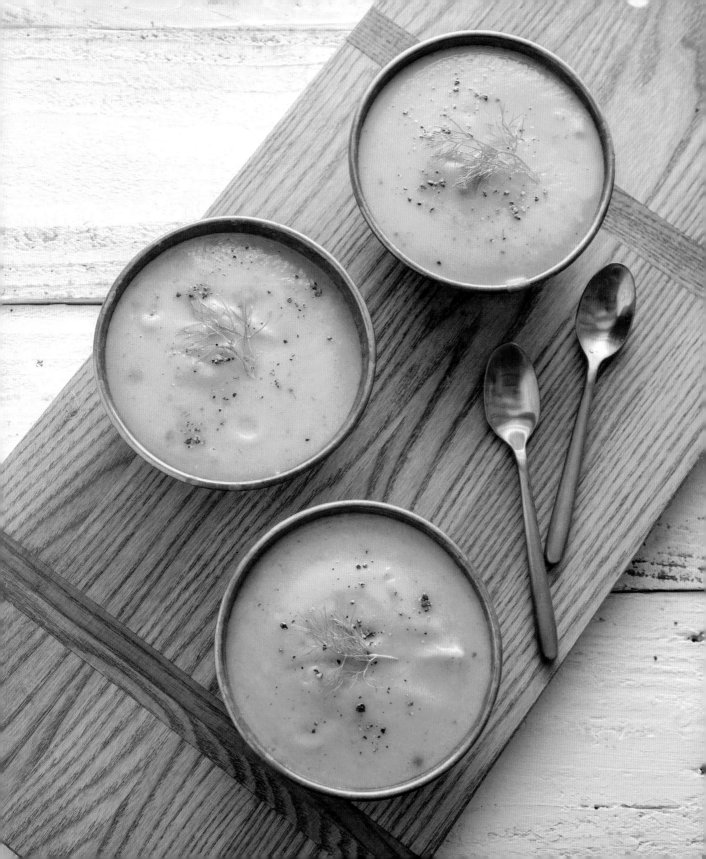

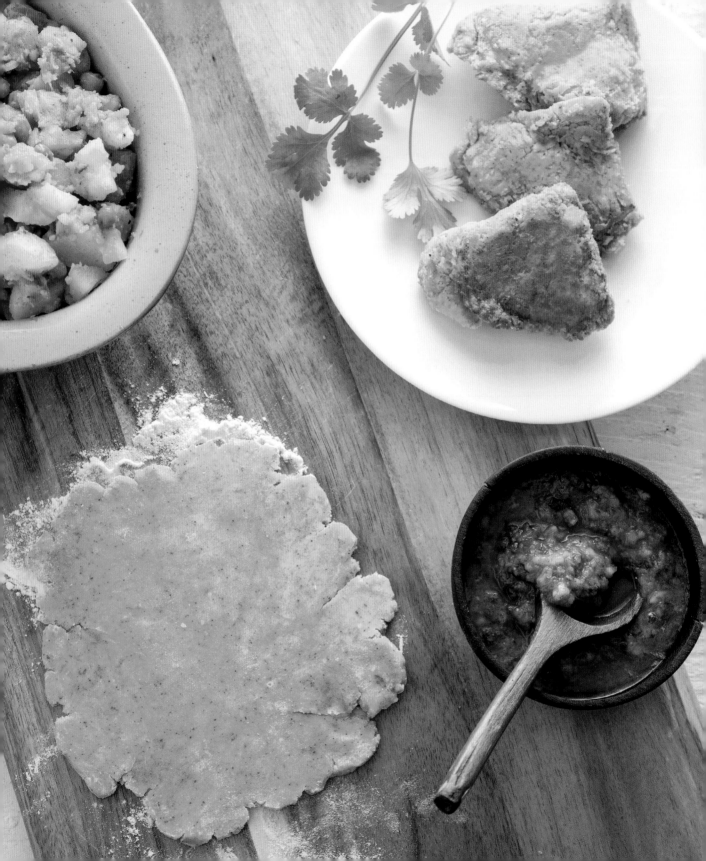

SWEET POTATO SAMOSA AND MANGO CHUTNEY
FOR FRIDAY

Sweet potato is unique among comfort foods for its ability to pacify. It is rich in beta-carotene, a Pitta-pacifying precursor to vitamin A.

YIELD: 4 servings

FOR THE DOUGH

1 cup (125 g) all-purpose flour, plus extra for kneading

¼ tsp paprika

¼ tsp salt

¼ tsp ground turmeric

1½ tbsp (22 g) coconut oil

1 tbsp (15 ml) water, plus more if needed

FOR THE CHUTNEY

8 oz (230 g) frozen mango, defrosted

1 tbsp (3 g) roughly chopped fresh mint

½ tbsp (2 g) roughly chopped fresh basil

Pinch of paprika

Salt, as desired

FOR THE FILLING

1 small sweet potato

1 small gold potato

¼ cup (30 g) fresh or frozen peas, defrosted

½ tsp ground cumin

¼ tsp ground cardamom

⅛ tsp garam masala

Salt, as desired

FOR THE SAMOSAS

1 cup (220 g) coconut oil, for frying

To make the dough, in a bowl, mix together the flour, paprika, salt and turmeric. Add the coconut oil and water. Mix until the dough comes together in a ball. Transfer the dough ball to a floured surface and knead until it's smooth. Cover it with plastic wrap and set it aside.

To make the chutney, add the mango, mint, basil, paprika and salt to a food processor and pulse until it's almost smooth. Set it aside.

To make the filling, microwave the potatoes for 2 minutes on each side. When the potatoes are cool, peel and chop them. Place the potatoes in a bowl and add the peas, cumin, cardamom, garam masala and salt. Toss to mix them.

To make the samosas, take a golf-ball-size piece of dough, form it into a ball and roll it into a circle using a rolling pin. Cut the circle in half. Take one of the halves and make a cone. Wet the edges with water and stick the edges together.

While holding a cone, add 1 tablespoon (20 g) of filling, wet one edge and pinch it together to seal.

Repeat until all the samosas are made.

In a large saucepan, heat the coconut oil in a large saucepan. Working in batches of four, fry the samosas for 5 minutes, or until golden brown. Drain them on paper towels and serve with the mango chutney.

Dosha Adaptations

This is a great tridoshic meal for the whole family!

SAMPLE KAPHA MEAL PLAN AND RECIPES

Shopping List

Meat and Seafood

- 6 boneless, skinless chicken thighs
- 3 cups (420 g) cooked and cubed chicken
- 1 chicken carcass

Vegetables and Fruit

- 4 acorn squashes
- 1 bell pepper
- 2 carrots
- 1 head cauliflower
- 1 celery stalk
- 1 lb (455 g) cremini mushrooms
- 1 garlic bulb
- 1 small ginger root
- ½ lb (230 g) green beans
- 1 jalapeño pepper
- 12 cups (804 g) chopped kale
- 2 leeks
- 1 lemon
- 1 lime
- 1 handful mint, 1 bunch basil, 1 bunch cilantro and 1 handful chives
- 4 yellow onions
- 1 handful parsley
- 2 sweet potatoes

Bakery and Miscellaneous

- 2 tbsp (16 g) arrowroot starch
- 1 (14-oz [400-g]) can artichoke hearts
- Cornbread
- ½ cup (65 g) dried cranberries (no sugar added)
- 2 tsp (10 g) dairy-free pesto
- ¼ cup (65 g) pumpkin or almond seed butter
- Pepper crackers
- ½ cup (70 g) raw pumpkin seeds
- 3 tbsp (45 ml) tamari
- 2 tbsp (30 g) tomato paste

Dairy

- 12 eggs
- Goat cheese

Pantry Staples

You may have these in your pantry, but if not, this is what you will need each week.

- Ajwan
- Apple cider vinegar
- Barley
- Basmati rice
- Black beans
- Buckwheat
- Canola oil
- Chickpeas
- Corn oil
- Corn tortillas
- Cornmeal
- Ghee
- Honey, raw and unprocessed
- Kidney beans
- Lentils
- Millet
- Oregano
- Quinoa
- Raisins
- Raw cane sugar
- Red lentils
- Rice milk
- Spices: asafetida, bay leaves, black pepper, cardamom, cayenne, chili powder, cinnamon, cloves, coriander, cumin, curry powder, fennel, fenugreek, mustard seeds, nutmeg, red pepper flakes, rosemary, saffron, salt, thyme, turmeric
- Sunflower oil
- Tofu
- Vegetable broth
- White beans

LENTIL-STUFFED SQUASH AND GRAVY
FOR MONDAY

The insoluble fiber found in lentils helps increase stool bulk and prevents a sluggish digestion, making this recipe great for detoxification.

YIELD: 4-6 servings

FOR THE STUFFED SQUASH

4 medium acorn squashes

2 tbsp (30 ml) sunflower oil

2½ cups (600 ml) vegetable broth

1 cup (200 g) dry green lentils, soaked overnight and rinsed

1 tbsp (15 ml) extra-virgin olive oil

2 cloves garlic, minced (optional)

1 small onion, finely diced (optional)

1 bell pepper, diced

2 carrots, finely diced or grated

1 celery rib, finely diced

1 heaping tsp dried thyme

½ heaping tsp cumin

Salt and pepper, as desired

FOR THE VEGETABLE GRAVY

2 tbsp (30 ml) sunflower oil

1 cup (160 g) diced yellow onion

2 cloves garlic, minced

1 lb (455 g) baby bella mushrooms, thinly sliced

2 cups (480 ml) vegetable broth or filtered water

3 tbsp (45 ml) low-sodium tamari

¾ tsp minced fresh thyme

2 tbsp (16 g) arrowroot or tapioca starch

Salt and pepper, as desired

Preheat the oven to 400°F (200°C).

To make the stuffed squash, cut the acorn squashes in half. Brush them thinly with the sunflower oil. Place them on a baking sheet and roast for 40 minutes, or until fork tender.

In a large pot, add the broth and the lentils. Bring it to a boil, reduce the heat, cover and simmer for about 40 minutes, or until the lentils are soft. Remove the lid and set the pot aside to cool, but do not drain it. The lentils will thicken a bit upon standing.

In a saucepan, heat the olive oil over medium heat. Sauté the garlic, onion, bell pepper, carrots and celery for about 5 minutes, or until the vegetables begin to soften. Add the thyme, cumin, salt and pepper, mixing well to incorporate them. Set it aside to cool.

Combine the sautéed vegetables with the lentils and mix well. Taste it, adding salt and pepper or any other herb or spice you might like, as needed.

To make the gravy, heat the sunflower oil in a saucepan over medium heat. Add the onion and garlic and sauté, stirring frequently, for about 4 minutes. Stir in the mushrooms and sauté until the mushrooms are tender, 5 to 6 minutes. Add the vegetable broth, tamari and thyme. Bring the mixture to a boil, lower the heat and simmer, covered, stirring occasionally, for 25 minutes, or until it thickens. Stir in the arrowroot and cook for 5 minutes. Transfer the gravy to a blender and puree it for a smooth consistency. Season with salt and pepper.

Spoon the vegetable lentil mixture into the squash halves. Top with the vegetable gravy.

Dosha Adaptations

This is a great tridoshic meal for the whole family!

WILD LEEK BAKED FRITTATA FOR TUESDAY

Packed with veggies, this frittata makes a well-rounded meal for breakfast, lunch or supper. Leeks contain the stress-reducing bioflavonoid quercetin, while oregano is deliciously antimicrobial and artichokes gently sustain liver functions.

YIELD: 6 servings

1 tsp extra-virgin olive oil

12 eggs

2 tsp (10 g) pesto

1 tsp dried thyme

1 tsp dried oregano

½ tsp sea salt

2 cups (178 g) finely chopped leeks (include greens)

1 (14-oz [400-g]) can artichoke hearts (packed in water), drained

1 cup (110 g) green beans, ends trimmed, cut into thirds

Crackers, for serving

Preheat the oven to 350°F (180°C). Grease a medium casserole dish with the olive oil and set it aside.

In a large bowl, whisk the eggs, pesto, thyme, oregano and salt and pour it into the oiled casserole dish. Layer it with the leeks, artichoke hearts and green beans. Bake for 30 minutes, or until the eggs are set. Serve hot with crackers.

Dosha Adaptations

PITTA: Add chapatis (unleavened flatbread) and ghee instead of crackers.
VATA: Replace the crackers with wheat rolls and ghee.

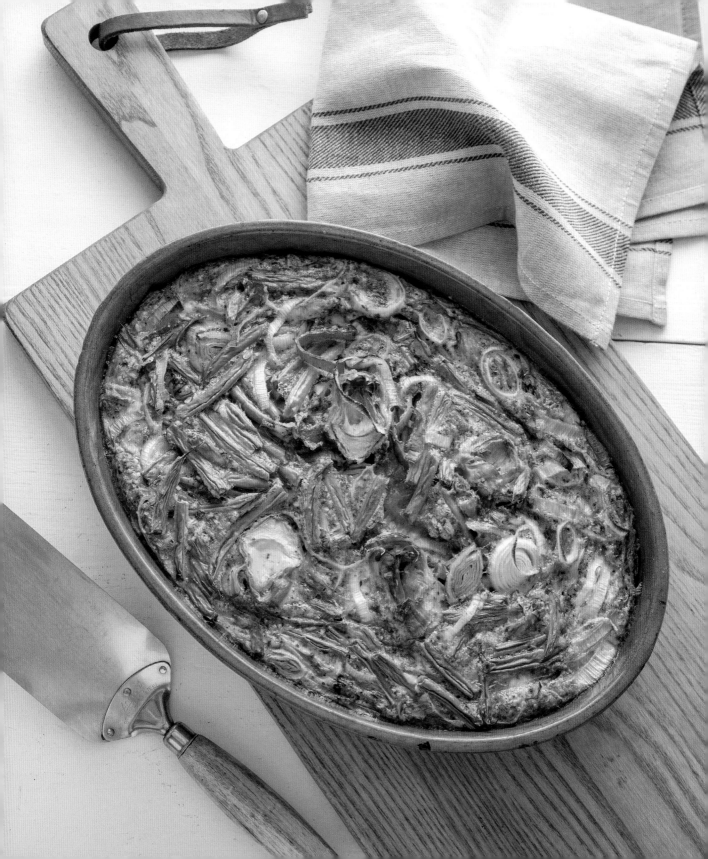

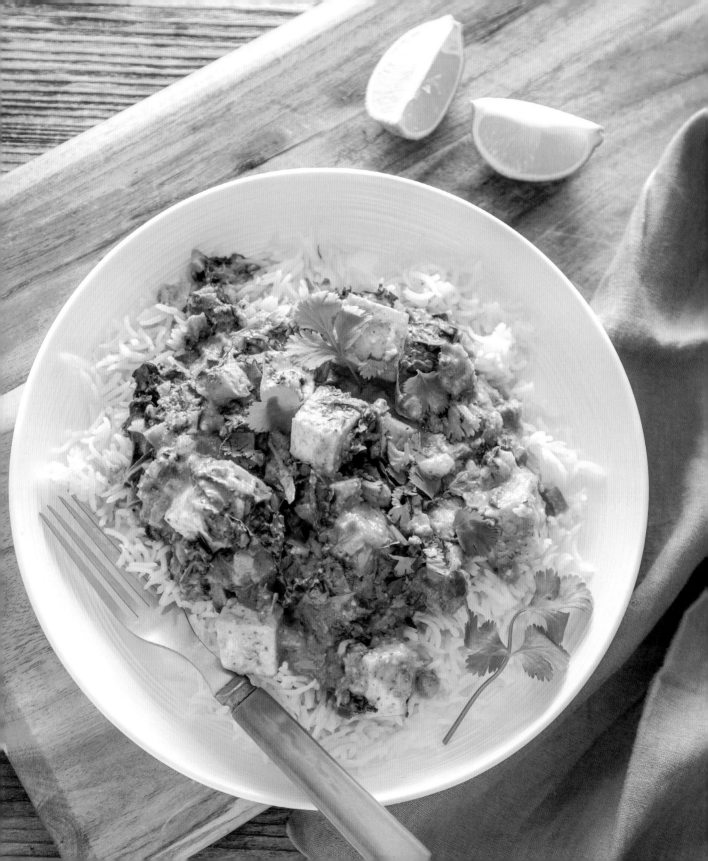

SPICY THAI BRAISED KALE AND TOFU
FOR WEDNESDAY

Ginger is known as a universal medicine benefiting everybody and all diseases. Especially good for Kapha disorders, this is one of Ayurveda's best go-to spices. When using ginger, think digestion, lungs and circulation, all Kapha problems.

YIELD: 2 servings

1 lb (455 g) extra-firm tofu, drained and cubed

½ cup (70 g) finely chopped onion

2 tbsp (18 g) grated fresh ginger

1 small jalapeño pepper, seeded and minced

2 tsp (6 g) cumin powder

2 cups (480 ml) vegetable broth

⅓ cup (85 g) unsalted almond butter

2 tbsp (30 g) tomato paste

Sea salt, as desired

1 bunch kale, stems removed and leaves chopped

1 tbsp (15 ml) fresh lime juice

1 large handful cilantro, chopped

2 cups (372 g) cooked rice

Preheat the oven to 350°F (180°C). Lightly oil a baking dish.

Place the tofu on the baking dish and bake for 15 minutes. Turn the tofu and bake for 15 minutes longer, or until lightly browned.

Heat a large saucepan and add the onion, ginger and jalapeño. Cook for 5 to 8 minutes, or until the onion has softened. Add the cumin and cook for 1 minute. Whisk in the vegetable broth, almond butter, tomato paste and salt and bring it to a boil. Gradually add the kale, stirring to let it wilt down. Add the baked tofu, cover, reduce the heat and simmer for 15 minutes, or until the kale is tender. Stir in the lime juice and cilantro. Serve over a bed of cooked rice.

Dosha Adaptations

PITTA: Pittas will need to add a yogurt raita to cool down this meal. Add 1 tablespoon (3 g) fresh mint to 4 tablespoons (60 g) of yogurt to make a yogurt raita.

VATA: Excellent dish for Vatas, especially if you add 1 teaspoon of ghee to the veggies.

CHICKEN KALE TURMERIC SOUP
FOR THURSDAY

Can chicken soup really cure a cold? I won't go so far as to claim it's a miracle healer, but I will say that a good chicken soup can boost your immune system and improve your chances of beating a virus. Turmeric is good at drying dampness and moving stagnation in the blood. It is a pungent, bitter and astringent herb that has a heating effect. It reduces excess Kapha and works specifically on the digestive, circulatory, respiratory and female reproductive systems.

YIELD: 5 servings

1 whole chicken carcass, stripped of meat

12 cups (3 L) water

1 rosemary sprig

¼ cup (60 ml) apple cider vinegar

Salt, as desired

2 large onions, chopped

1 large bay leaf

1 tbsp (9 g) turmeric powder

3 cups (420 g) chopped organic chicken meat

3 cups (200 g) chopped kale

4 cloves garlic, grated

2 tbsp (18 g) grated ginger

In a large pot, add the chicken carcass, water, rosemary, apple cider vinegar and salt and bring it to a boil over high heat. Reduce the heat to a simmer and stir well. Cover it and cook for 2 hours. Strain the soup to remove the solids and return the liquid to the pot. Add the onions, bay leaf and turmeric. Bring it to a boil and cook for 10 minutes.

Add the chopped chicken and simmer for approximately 10 minutes, or until the flavors meld. Stir in the kale, garlic and ginger. Simmer for another 2 minutes to blend the flavors and cook the kale. Remove the bay leaf and serve.

Dosha Adaptations

PITTA: Serve with some sunflower seed crackers and ghee.
VATA: Serve with warm wheat rolls and ghee.

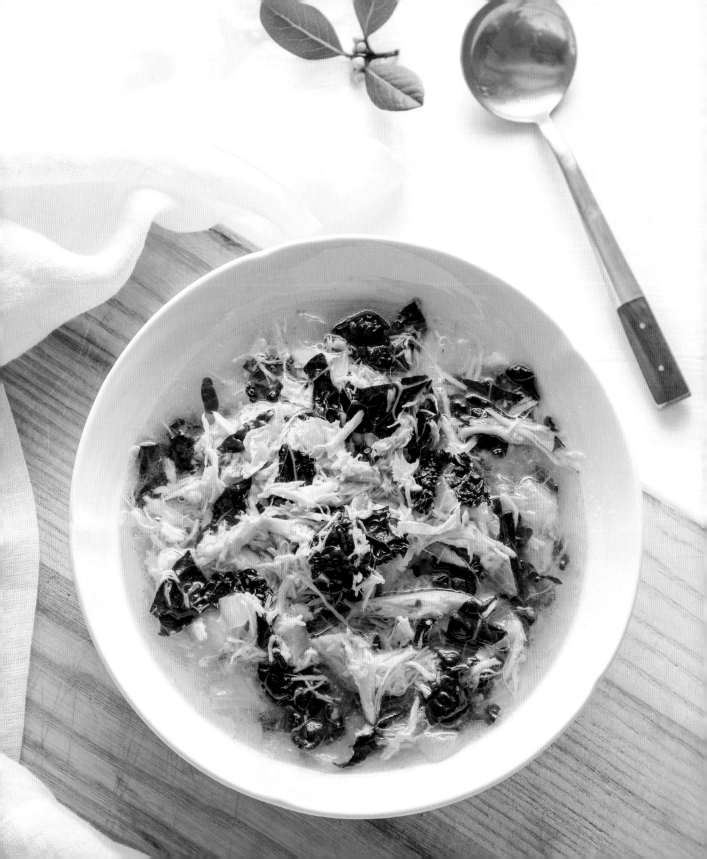

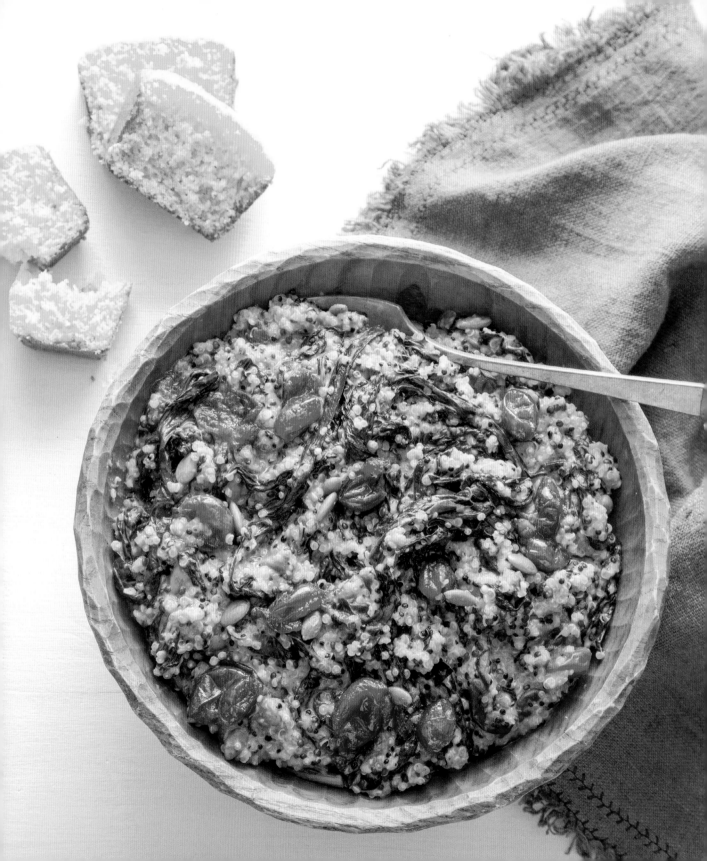

QUINOA KALE CRANBERRY SALAD
FOR FRIDAY

Easy to prepare, easy to digest and nutrient-dense, quinoa is a simple, practical and straightforward choice for everyone. The super-food has earned its place alongside hall-of-fame staples like kale, brown rice and broccoli. Quinoa can help curb carb cravings and maintain a healthy weight. Often carbohydrate and sugar cravings are protein cravings in disguise. If you crave carbs, which Kaphas often do, make quinoa your first choice.

YIELD: 4 servings

FOR THE DRESSING

¼ cup (65 g) almond butter

¼ cup (60 ml) apple cider

Juice from ½ lemon

½ tsp sea salt or pink rock salt

FOR THE QUINOA

1 cup (180 g) uncooked quinoa

2½ cups (600 ml) water, divided

8 cups (536 g) kale, stems removed, cut into ribbons

½ cup (70 g) raw pumpkin seeds

½ cup (65 g) dried no-sugar-added cranberries

Cornbread, warmed, for serving

For the dressing, in a bowl combine the almond butter, apple cider, lemon juice and salt. Set it aside.

For the quinoa, in a medium pot, place the quinoa and 1½ cups (360 ml) of the water. Bring it to a boil, reduce the heat and simmer for 15 minutes, covered. Remove the pot from the heat, let it sit for 5 minutes, then fluff the quinoa with a fork and let it cool.

In a large pot, place the kale and the remaining 1 cup (240 ml) of water. Bring it to a boil, turn off the heat and cover. Let it steam for 2 minutes, or until the kale is soft. Drain well. Add the quinoa, pumpkin seeds and cranberries. Mix well to combine them. Serve warm with cornbread.

Dosha Adaptations

PITTA: Serve with hot chapatis and ghee instead of cornbread, and raisins instead of cranberries.

VATA: Serve with chapatis instead of cornbread, and dates instead of cranberries.

KEEP THE GOOD THINGS WORKING IN YOUR LIFE

Remember that the key to moving on with vitality and health is balance. Working on decreasing the habits that are not so great while working on sustainable changes slowly will be really worth it for you.

I see today that a lot of people are deeply disillusioned with the kind of quick-fix mentality you find in conventional medicine. And millions are turning to complementary and alternative forms of medicine, which tend to tap into a slower and gentler holistic form of healing. It is clearly unique in this day and age to find a system of medicine that is more than five thousand years old and still one of the largest on the planet. Although Ayurveda is in its infancy here in the United States, it has more than three hundred thousand physicians worldwide, making it one of the largest medical organizations in the world.

Perhaps the reason for Ayurveda's longevity is its simple and clear definition of health: a state of a balanced mind, a well-formed body and good elimination. When the doshas are in balance, when the mind and body are in harmony, only then is optimal health achieved.

This is what I help people attain, and this is what I can help *you* with. Please join us on the Holistic Highway blog and sign up to be part of the Holistic Highway community. Interacting with a supportive community is so important to building your new, healthier life. Please know that you are welcome to join us online or in person.

I hope that this book helps guide you to a new and healthy life. Stay true to the following nine behaviors and you will maintain the great changes you have already made:

- Wake up before sunrise.
- Have a nutritious breakfast according to your dosha.
- Have your biggest meal of the day at lunch.
- Never eat and run!
- Eat freshly cooked or prepared meals.
- Take at least 20 minutes a day just for yourself.
- Turn off electronics at least 1 hour before bed.
- Go to bed between 10:00 and 11:00 p.m.
- Do a seasonal cleanse.

HEALTH TRACKER AND FOOD LOG

The health tracker chart and food log will help you keep track of what you eat, how you feel, how much you exercise and how much you sleep. Make copies so you can fill in the charts and notice any changes before they become problematic.

Health Tracker

1 Being Low and 10 Being the Best You Ever Felt

		1-3	4-7	8-10	COMMENTS
EMOTIONS	M				
	T				
	W				
	T				
	F				
	S				
	S				
SLEEPING	M				
	T				
	W				
	T				
	F				
	S				
	S				
ENERGY LEVELS	M				
	T				
	W				
	T				
	F				
	S				
	S				
EXERCISE	M				
	T				
	W				
	T				
	F				
	S				
	S				

Food Log

BREAKFAST	LUNCH	DINNER	SNACKS
MONDAY			
TUESDAY			
WEDNESDAY			
THURSDAY			
FRIDAY			
SATURDAY			
SUNDAY			

FAQS

To help you further with the concepts of this cleanse and to help you with any challenges you may have going forward, let me share with you some of the questions I get from others like you who have gone through the cleanse.

Q: I am worried about constipation. Can I take a laxative on the cleanse?

A: Laxatives actually encourage your system to stop working naturally as the laxative does the job for you. Laxatives will irritate the colon, and while they will help you go, ultimately they will dry out the GI tract. Use the triphala (page 37) to help improve peristalsis.

Q: I am worried I will get hungry between meals. What can I snack on?

A: One of the most important strategies of the Ayurveda cleanse is to ignite your digestive fire (metabolism). Your body cannot do that without some intermittent fasting. It is recommended you refrain from snacking between meals; however, you can drink warm water. As your blood sugar stabilizes and your digestion becomes more efficient, your need for snacks will decrease.

Q: I am concerned about caffeine withdrawal. What can I do about headaches I normally get when coming off caffeine?

A: You may suffer a headache as your body detoxifies. This will pass as you go through the pre-cleanse. Try tapering off caffeine and sugar. So, for example, if you are used to drinking 3 cups (720 ml) of coffee a day, reduce your cups by one for a couple of days, and then by another and then finally, drink ½ cup (120 ml) before coming off altogether. Also, drink plenty of water and your detox tea (page 31).

Q: Can I use decaf coffee?

A: It is not recommended, as decaf coffee still has some caffeine, and depending upon how it has been decaffeinated, it can add more chemicals to your body.

Q: I have increased my water content so much that I have to get up constantly during the night. What can I do?

A: Stop drinking water by 7:00 p.m. In other words, drink your water during the day.

Q: Am I getting enough protein on this cleanse?

A: We think we need more protein than we actually do. The Ayurveda cleanse offers more than enough protein and fiber; however, you can always add some hemp, rice or pea protein if you feel the need.

Q: Shall I stop taking my medications on the Ayurveda cleanse?

A: No, continue taking all your prescribed medications. If you are unsure if the Ayurveda cleanse is for you, please check with your physician.

Q: I would prefer to use applesauce instead of raw apples. Is there any problem with that?

A: Try eating the fresh apples as the whole apple is what will help in the pre-cleanse with the bile and liver. However, you can use malic acid if apples disagree with you.

Q: I don't like the taste of water. Can I add some flavor?

A: No, it is better to use plain filtered water.

Q: On the pre-cleanse, there is a lot of food, and I cannot get through it all. I just feel stuffed.

A: Just eat until you are no longer hungry. There is no point in plowing through your food just because it is there. Eat until you are satiated, but do eat enough to see you through to the next meal.

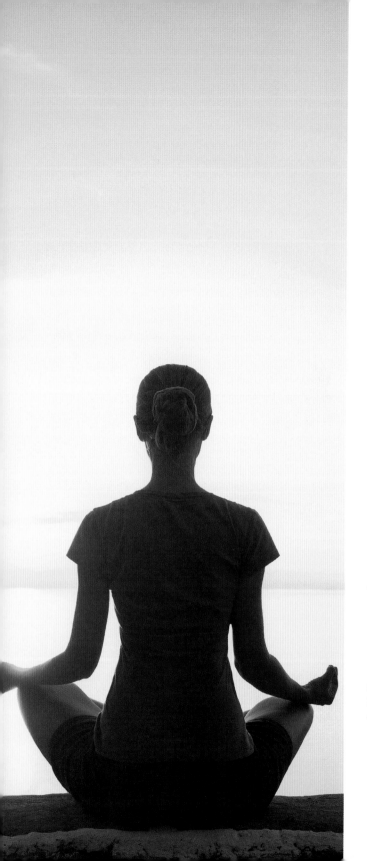

Q: I am a vegan and do not want to use animal products. What can I use instead of ghee?

A: You can use sesame oil.

Q: I prefer ice in my water. Why can't I have iced water?

A: Ice in your water will slow down digestive enzymes and make digestion more difficult. That means you will not detoxify as well. Hang in there—you will come to love your warmer water over time.

Q: I am an active person and am considering training for a marathon or other significant event. Is it okay for me to cleanse?

A: I would advise that this is not a good time for you to cleanse. All cleanses are somewhat depleting—it is a time to take a step back from intensive exercise and training routines. I would suggest shorter workouts and practicing the yoga sequences for each phase.

Q: I am pregnant. Can I cleanse?

A: No, this cleanse would not be good to do while pregnant or while breast-feeding. Pregnant women and nursing mothers have very unique nutritional needs. If you have any questions, check with your physician.

Q: Can I use stevia on the cleanse?

A: It would be better to refrain from using sweeteners at the end of the pre-cleanse and during the cleanse. In the post-cleanse you can start adding back a sweetener.

For more information on what I do and to go a little deeper into how Ayurveda can be a blueprint for your health that you can use for the rest of your life, see my website at www.theholistichighway.com.

GLOSSARY

Abhyanga (AH-bee-young-ga): A full-body oil massage that's done from head to toe.

Agni (ahg-nee): Our digestive fire; governs our metabolism.

Ama (ah-ma): Fat soluble toxins that are formed in the body due to poor digestion and imbalances.

Ayurveda (eye-your-vay-da): The science of life or the science of longevity; the world's oldest system of medicine based upon balancing the body, mind and soul.

Dosha (doe-sha): One of the three metabolic types (Vata, Pitta and Kapha) that are made up of the five great elements.

Ghee (gee): Clarified butter used in a prebiotic cleanse because of its cooling and nourishing properties.

Kapalabhati (kar-pal-bha-tee): A type of breathwork that uses continuous expirations.

Kapha (kar-far): The dosha or metabolic type that brings lubrication, structure and strength to the body. Made of the elements earth and water.

Kitchari (kit-char-ee): Ayurveda's superfood. A simple digestible meal of mung beans and rice that helps with digestion and is used in the heart of the cleanse.

Nadi Shodhanam (nar-dee-show-da-num): A type of pranayama featuring alternate nostril breathing. Used to calm and ground the nervous system

Nasya (nars-ya): An herbalized oil applied to the nose via drops to clean and lubricate the mucous membranes of the nasal passages.

Ojas (oh-jus): That essence of our health we know as vitality and translates to physical immunity.

Pitta (pit-ah): The dosha or metabolic type that brings transformations and change to the body. Made of the elements fire and water.

Pranayama (prahn-nu-yarm-ah): A therapeutic type of breathwork often called yogic breathwork.

Sanskrit (sans-krit): An ancient vibrational language that Ayurveda was written in.

Trikatu (tri-ka-tu): An herbal remedy made from three peppers. It supports the digestive system.

Triphala (tri-fal-la): An herbal remedy made from three fruits. It tones the digestive system.

Vata (vart-uh): The dosha or metabolic type that brings movement to the body. Made of the elements air and space.

Vipaka (vi-pah-kha): The post-digestive effect of food.

Yoga (yo-gha): Means union.

RESOURCES

AYURVEDA CENTERS

The Holistic Highway meal plan
theholistichighway.com/ayurveda-recipe-program

The Holistic Highway blog
theholistichighway.com/blog

The Holistic Highway private Facebook Group
facebook.com/groups/951807431497157

The Chopra Center
chopra.com

The Ayurvedic Institute
ayurveda.com

John Douillard's LifeSpa
lifespa.com

AYURVEDA HERBS

Banyan Botanicals
banyanbotanicals.com

VPK by Maharishi Ayurveda
mapi.com

AYURVEDA ORGANIZATIONS

National Ayurvedic Medical Association (NAMA)
ayurvedanama.org

Association of Ayurvedic Professionals of North America (AAPNA)
aapna.org

ESSENTIAL OILS

Floracopeia
floracopeia.com

Nature's Oil
naturesoil.com

VIDEO DEMONSTRATIONS

Go to the Holistic Highway YouTube channel for links to videos about agni, making ghee, daily exercises and more.

https://www.youtube.com/channel/UCp7I9qjjdE4PE-0OVJEop5QQ/videos

If you would like to join me with your yoga or meditation, go to www.theholistichighway.com/bookspecial and type in the password "Ayurveda." Here you'll find videos and audio to accompany the book, and we can do this together.

ACKNOWLEDGMENTS

The world is a better place thanks to people who guide and help others. What makes it even better are people who share the gift of Ayurveda to teach future health leaders. Thank you to those that have come before me, whose legacies I stand on to grow and help others grow. It would not have been possible without you, my Ayurveda family, including: Dr. Vasant Lad, whose humble teachings resonate deep inside me; Dr. John Douillard, who taught me to look at the science; Dr. Claudia Welch, who showed me that all systems of medicine are connected; Baba Ji who took me deep into Ayurveda psychology; Hilary Garivaltis, who I still remember saying with great kindness on my first day of class, "If you are going to study Ayurveda, then you need to know how to pronounce it"; and my first tribe, Kripalu, and my second tribe, Om My Yoga. This book is a combination of all your teachings.

Writing a book is harder than I thought and more rewarding than I could have ever imagined. None of this would have been possible without my best friend, and sister, Sally. She has been my biggest cheerleader and has stood by me during every struggle and all my successes. That is true friendship . . . and family. Thank you.

To my son and business partner, Justin, for believing we should build an Ayurveda company based upon integrity, science and a genuine desire to guide people onto the road to health.

To my friend Michelle, who often said, "You still have to eat!" and would show up with home-cooked soup. I may have starved without you. To Melissa, whose ongoing support is priceless and who is quietly there, offering the words "How can I help?" We have come a long way, baby, haven't we?!

To my colleagues at the University of Pittsburgh Center for Integrative Medicine. To be part of such an awesome team is indeed awe-inspiring.

Thanks to everyone at Page Street Publishing who has helped me so much. A special thanks to my editors Sarah Monroe and Karen Levy, who with immense patience have helped me hone the most important aspects of an Ayurveda cleanse and turn it into this beautiful book. I also want to give a huge shout-out to Toni Zernik, who took my recipes, actually cooked them herself and showcased them in such a way as to make them look exquisite. You are a true artist.

And lastly, to Bailey, my dog, who made sure I took time out of writing this book to walk and roughhouse. Thank you for reminding me that all work has to be balanced with play and that sometimes just sitting in the sun cures all ills.

ABOUT THE AUTHOR

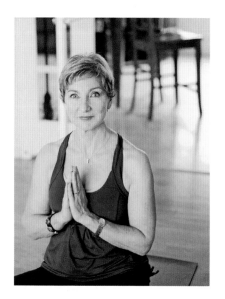

KERRY HARLING'S ethos as a health professional is that health is NOT one size fits all. Each of us is unique, and as such requires individualized treatment. Her philosophy on health and medicine began when, as part of her graduate studies, she observed the effects of environmental toxins on human health, toxins that left patients with a myriad of symptoms that didn't have a specific diagnosis. She has since dedicated her life to developing an integrative approach to medicine that combines the individualized approach of Ayurveda with the benefits of modern technology, such as genetics. Working within the field of epigenetics, she combines the wisdom of Eastern medicine with the breakthroughs of Western technology, and is able to create wellness plans for her patients that are personalized down to the molecular level.

Kerry has a B.S. in neuroscience, a master's degree in education and has studied at the Kripalu School of Ayurveda and the world-renowned Ayurvedic Institute. She is CEO of the Holistic Highway where she helps her clients achieve optimal health through customized health services and programs. She also has a practice at the University of Pittsburgh's Center for Integrative Medicine, runs the Ayurveda Sanctuary, is a registered practitioner with the National Ayurvedic Medical Association (NAMA), is a certified yoga teacher and is the creator of the TEDx Talk "Context Is Everything."

RECIPE INDEX

GENERAL INDEX